WORKING WITH
LARYNGECTOMEES

Dedication

This book is dedicated to the laryngectomees who
have passed through Singleton Hospital as part of
their rehabilitation.

WORKING WITH
LARYNGECTOMEES

ERYL EVANS

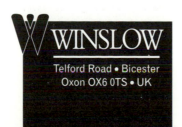

WINSLOW

Telford Road • Bicester
Oxon OX6 0TS • UK

First published in 1990 by
Winslow Press Limited, Telford Road, Bicester, Oxon OX6 OTS,
United Kingdom
Reprinted 1991, 1993, 1996

Phototypeset by Gecko Limited, Bicester, Oxon

02–854/Printed in Great Britain by Hobbs the Printers Limited,
Southampton

British Library Cataloguing in Publication Data
Evans, Eryl
  Working with laryngectomees.
  1. Laryngectomy patients. Rehabilitations
  I. Title
  617.533059

ISBN 0–86388–083–5

CONTENTS

Eryl Evans MCST, LCST

Eryl Evans qualified as a speech therapist from the Cardiff School of Speech Therapy in 1978. After working as a general therapist in North Wales she moved in 1980 to a specialist post at Singleton Hospital, Swansea, which gave her the opportunity to work intensively with voice disorders and laryngectomees.

In 1986 she attended the Mayo Clinic Laryngectomee Rehabilitation Seminar in Honolulu, and in the same year contributed a chapter to the book edited by Fawcus, *Voice Disorders and their Management*. She completed the College of Speech Therapists' Advanced Specialist Course in Voice Disorders in 1988.

She is at present Head of Adult Services for West Glamorgan Health Authority, and a visiting lecturer at the Cardiff School of Speech Therapy.

FOREWORD

In her introduction to this text, Eryl Evans clearly defines her aim in compiling this book – to provide clinicians with practical management and therapeutic suggestions for assisting laryngectomees at different stages of rehabilitation. In fact, this book covers much more than this modest aim. Eryl has provided the most up-to-date information, including a comprehensive section on Surgical Voice Restoration (notably the Blom–Singer procedure) which will greatly assist clinicians new to this technique who may be lacking in knowledge and in confidence. Although the book is filled with accurate detail and helpful suggestions, the atmosphere pervading the text is one of sympathy and sensitivity towards the patient.

Since Gaye Murrills attended the Mayo Clinic Laryngectomee Rehabilitation Seminar in 1977, and Yvonne Edels followed in 1979, therapists in this country have attempted to promote laryngectomee rehabilitation in the United Kingdom by introducing modern practices learnt there. Eryl has joined this group by using her training at the Mayo Clinic to introduce Surgical Voice Restoration at her own hospital in Swansea and to produce this helpful and practical management book.

The chapter on pre-operative visiting gives accurate and sensible advice for the clinician to follow and the issues which may arise at this time are covered sensitively and sympathetically. Wherever possible, advice is followed with references to the literature and this helps the clinician who wishes to read further into the subject. Following in a logical progression, from pre-operative visit to post-operative therapy and even a discussion of the role of the clinician in terminal care, Eryl shows a sensible and practical approach in her suggestions, and her experience in laryngectomy is evident from the text. The much-needed section on evaluation and assessment for Surgical Voice Restoration and the clarity of the illustrations in the text should make this area of laryngectomee rehabilitation now accessible for any clinician who is undertaking this work.

The check-lists, illustrations and suggestions for word lists should mean that, at last, clinicians in this field have a way of annotating and formally assessing clients' progress. The constant emphasis, throughout the text, on measuring and assessing progress will be appreciated by all clinicians who are interested in quality assurance, especially those inexperienced in this field.

Eryl is to be congratulated on producing such a clear, comprehensive, practical text which will be of use both to new therapists working with laryngectomees and those who wish to be brought up-to-date with the newer surgical techniques. I predict that this will become a standard work in clinics where laryngectomees are treated; it is a much-needed and welcome addition to the field.

Alison Perry
1990

ACKNOWLEDGEMENTS

I would like to thank family, friends and colleagues for their guidance and encouragement, without which this book could not have been written.

Special thanks are due to Sheila Edwards for the illustrations, Julie Jones for help with typing, and Sally Eakins and Marilyn Morgan for their unfailing encouragement over many months. Along with Stephanie Martin, calmly editing the text, their support has been invaluable, and I welcome this opportunity to thank them.

CHAPTER 1
INTRODUCTION

CHAPTER 1
INTRODUCTION

Working with laryngectomees can be one of the most rewarding aspects of rehabilitation, but it can also cause clinicians great anxiety if they have little experience of working with this client group.

The aim of this book is to provide clinicians with practical management and therapeutic suggestions for dealing with laryngectomees at different stages of their rehabilitation. It does not aim to replace standard textbooks, which may provide more detailed information about aspects of laryngectomee rehabilitation outside the scope of this book. The reader is referred to the bibliography for a list of these.

The contents are set out in what would be the usual sequence of management, although there are no rigid rules. *Chapter 2* deals with the anatomical and physiological aspects of dealing with the laryngectomee pre- and post-operatively. Often the patient is keen to know more about what is going to happen during surgery. Clinicians too need to be aware of the specific details of the procedure.

Chapter 3 discusses the benefits of the pre-operative visit, and outlines a suggested format for dealing with this visit.

Chapter 4 discusses the first post-operative visit, describing different circumstances in which it may occur, depending on when the patient is first referred.

Chapter 5 describes oesophageal voice, what it is, and stages which may be helpful in therapy aimed at establishing oesophageal voice as the laryngectomee's method of communication.

Where oesophageal voice is not developed easily, there may be many and varied reasons – some easily remedied, others more difficult. *Chapter 6* discusses some of these difficulties and outlines suggested means of dealing with them.

Chapter 7 discusses the application of communication aids – specifically the artificial larynx – when working with laryngectomees. Some of the different aids available are described, along with suggested programmes of therapy.

In recent years, surgical innovations have been developed to try and overcome the problems of the laryngectomy removing the source of voice production. *Chapters 8* and *9* discuss present trends in Surgical Voice Restoration, and outline ways in which the clinician may be involved in the voice rehabilitation team.

Chapter 10 is a collection of various 'extra' information which may be useful when dealing with laryngectomees and, along with *Chapter 11*, suggests various resources and sources of information for the clinician.

CHAPTER 2
ANATOMY & PHYSIOLOGY

CHAPTER 2
ANATOMY &
PHYSIOLOGY

Introduction

The surgical procedures involved in carrying out a laryngectomy change the structures of the head and neck area completely. The mechanisms of swallowing and therefore eating and drinking, as well as phonation, are affected and it is essential that the clinician has a clear idea of the anatomy and physiology of the patient pre- and post-operatively. This is in order to explain it to the patient and family, and so that the procedures and their implications are clear in the clinician's mind.

This chapter describes pre- and post-operative anatomical structures and also outlines the surgical procedures involved in laryngectomy. Precise surgical details should, however, be ascertained from discussion with the surgeon involved, as preferred techniques vary from surgeon to surgeon, from area to area, as well as from patient to patient. Surgical and healing details will also be affected by whether radiotherapy has taken place pre-operatively, or is to take place post-operatively, and these details should also be checked.

Pre-operative Anatomy

The structures involved in swallowing and phonation are shown in *Figure 1*, and this diagram can be used with the patient when discussing the implications of surgery. The process of laryngeal phonation should be outlined, by describing the passage of air into the lungs via a completely open vocal tract, and out past the closed vocal folds, whose vibration produces voice. It is often useful during this discussion to explain that it is the articulators of the mouth and oropharynx which produce the speech sounds, and that the larynx is only responsible for the sound in speech. Some laryngectomees report fearing that speech as a whole would be taken away from them along with their larynx. (As clinicians, it is easy for us to forget that not everyone is as aware of the process of communication as we are.)

The process for phonation should be contrasted with that for swallowing, where the passage of the bolus of food into the stomach involves the same structures until it reaches the level of the larynx when the epiglottis protects the opening into the larynx, so that food does not pass into the trachea. In swallowing, the vocal folds form a secondary 'safety valve' preventing aspiration of food or liquids into the lungs.

Figure 1   **Pre-operative structure – vocal tract**

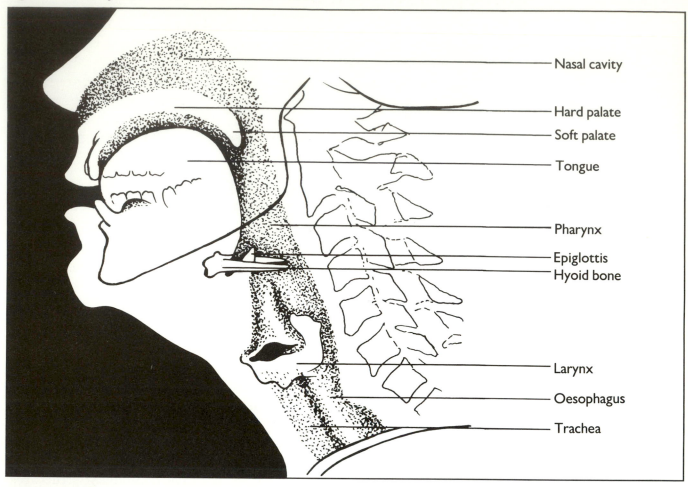

- Nasal cavity
- Hard palate
- Soft palate
- Tongue
- Pharynx
- Epiglottis
- Hyoid bone
- Larynx
- Oesophagus
- Trachea

Figure 2   **Post-laryngectomy vocal tract**

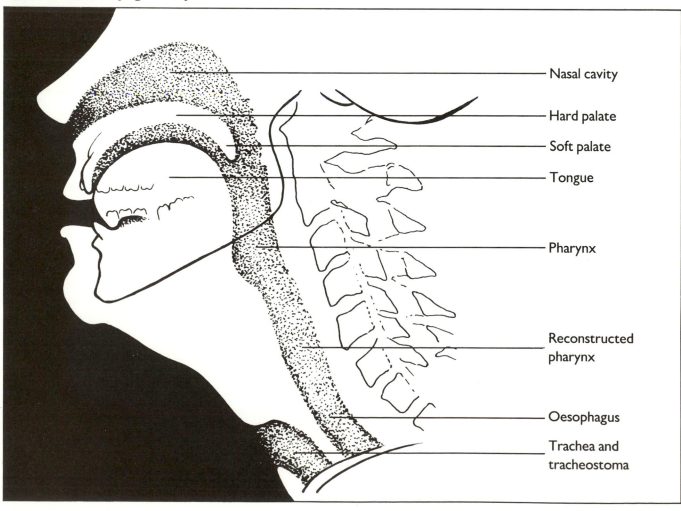

- Nasal cavity
- Hard palate
- Soft palate
- Tongue
- Pharynx
- Reconstructed pharynx
- Oesophagus
- Trachea and tracheostoma

Post-operative Anatomy

Following laryngectomy, the anatomy of the head and neck area can be represented by a diagram such as *Figure 2*, and again this can be used in discussion with the patient. The separate mechanisms for breathing and swallowing can be shown, as well as the alternatives for post-surgical phonation. The expected position of the pharyngo-oesophageal segment can be shown, with the patient becoming familiar with the terms associated with the procedure – tracheostoma, pharynx, oesophagus. Where Surgical Voice Restoration is being considered, the clinician is referred to the diagrams in *Chapter 8*.

Extent and Location of Tumour

The location of the tumour will have been investigated by indirect and direct laryngoscopy in most patients, and the extent of spread noted. **Berry** (1983) outlines the international system of tumour staging or classification. The laryngeal area is divided into supraglottic, glottic and subglottic regions as follows:

Supraglottis:
posterior surface of the suprahyoid epiglottis
aryepiglottic fold
arytenoid
epiglottis below the hyoid
ventricular bands
ventricular cavities
Glottis:
vocal cords (folds)
anterior commissure
posterior commissure
Subglottis:
all areas below the glottis

Laryngeal tumours are classified according to the extent of penetration into surrounding structures:

T_1 tumour: limited to the region of origin without affecting the mobility of the structure;
T_2 tumour: extends to surrounding region but vocal fold mobility is not affected;
T_3 tumour: limited to the larynx with one or both vocal folds immobile;
T_4 tumour: extends into surrounding structures beyond the larynx, eg. post-cricoid region, pyriform fossa.

Investigations will also have identified any palpable lymph glands which would suggest that the disease has spread to other tissues in the neck. The presence or absence of distant metastases – disease spreading further than the surrounding neck glands – would usually be noted where apparent.

Radiotherapy

In the United Kingdom the majority of patients presenting for laryngectomy will have had pre-operative radiotherapy, as compared with North America where surgery is usually the primary procedure. Therapeutic radiotherapy is successful in 80–90 per cent of cases (**Berry**, 1983) and in the remainder tumour size is reduced. Failure is usually associated with local recurrence too close to the irradiated area to permit further treatment. Post-operative radiotherapy may be necessary where disease spread is extensive, or where there is disease recurrence.

In general, radiotherapy can result in a decrease in tissue elasticity, which may cause problems in surgical procedures, or in later voice acquisition, but these occasional difficulties should not detract from the fact that a large percentage of patients with laryngeal disease can be spared laryngectomy by undergoing radiotherapy. In addition, conflicting research results (**Simpson** *et al.*, 1972; **Richardson**, 1981) regarding the effect of radiotherapy on voice acquisition suggest that radiotherapy should not automatically be seen as a hindrance to successful rehabilitation. Many clinicians will report vocal success with patients who have had large doses of radiation.

For further details the reader is referred to **Berry** (1983) for a comprehensive description of the techniques and procedures of radiotherapy in the United Kingdom.

Surgical Procedure

It has already been stated that surgical procedures will vary greatly, depending on the surgeon as well as the individual patient and the site and extent of the tumour. The successful removal of the life-threatening tumour, leaving a satisfactory clearance margin of healthy tissue, must be the surgeon's primary concern, followed by a safe, functional reconstruction of the pharynx.

The initial incision is made to give good exposure of the larynx and is often 'U-shaped', and may or may not accommodate the tracheostoma site. (The tracheostoma may be fashioned at a site slightly below the incision line.) Following division of the neck muscles, the larynx is exposed, and its blood supply ligated. The trachea may be cut at this stage and sutured to the neck to form the tracheostoma. As the initial endotracheal tube would pass through the surgical area it is usually removed at this stage, and anaesthesia continued via the newly formed tracheostoma.

The larynx is then removed, along with the hyoid bone and any lymph glands in the area, leaving an opening in the pharynx (the pharynx is attached to the back of the larynx). The amount of pharyngeal tissue removed is affected by the extent and spread of the tumour.

The pharyngeal mucosa is then closed and ease of closure is affected by the amount of tissue which has been removed. The pharyngeal muscles are then sutured carefully over the mucosa in several layers; there has been much discussion regarding the effects of different methods of muscle closure on acquisition of voice post-operatively (**Cheesman**, 1983, **Stafford**, 1989). Suction drains are placed in the neck to ensure that blood and other secretions do not collect and impede healing.

The necessity for neck dissection for removal of diseased lymph glands does not prolong surgery to a great extent, but can result in numbness of the surrounding tissues and problems with shoulder strength on the affected side.

Post-operative Appearance

Some laryngectomees may return from theatre with a laryngectomy tube in place, although this is not always so. (If the stoma is fashioned large enough, then a tube should not be necessary.) They may also have an intravenous feeding system, along with drainage tubes. On the ward they may be connected to a humidifier which ensures warm moist air is taken into the lungs through the tracheostoma. A nasogastric feeding tube may also have been inserted, although feeding via this is deferred until bowel movements recommence, usually 24 hours after surgery.

Extensive Surgery

The procedures outlined above refer to relatively uncomplicated laryngectomy, where the disease spread is not extensive. Where the tumour has spread into the post-cricoid region or pyriform fossa, then more extensive surgery may be necessary, and this has implications for the management of the patient. Procedures for ensuring a clear margin of disease-free tissue may involve the surgeon carrying out a pharyngo-laryngo-oesophagectomy, and reconstruction of the pharynx using a transplanted piece of colon, grafted skin tube, or by pulling up the stomach and anastomosing the fundus of the stomach to the pharynx.

Following extensive surgery, the clinician should expect a delay in full rehabilitation, and the use of a communication aid should be encouraged to ensure immediate effective communication. Often the prognosis for these patients is poor, and so delays in speech rehabilitation should be avoided.

CHAPTER 3
PRE-OPERATIVE VISIT

CHAPTER 3
PRE-OPERATIVE VISIT

Introduction

If it is at all possible, rehabilitation of the laryngectomee should not be delayed until convalescence is under way, or the laryngectomee is 'ready' post-operatively to commence therapy. It must be recognised that fear of the unknown can be a major cause of anxiety, and inadequate preparation for the surgery can result in a post-operative reaction which can affect rehabilitation.

There is still some discussion as to whether the patient should be totally informed pre-operatively, since they may refuse to undertake what is, essentially, life-saving surgery. It has been noted by **Pitkin** (1953), among others, that the 'post-operative emotional makeup of the individual' was influenced by the management and preparation pre-operatively.

In most cases, some pre-operative information is given to the prospective laryngectomee, with the patient being given as much or as little information as they can cope with. Even though the information may be given in a logical, straightforward manner, this does not guarantee comprehension and assimilation of the facts by the patient, as anxiety and fear can impede the amount of information that is assimilated.

The clinician and other staff involved in giving this information must be prepared both to repeat themselves and to modify the extent and depth of information according to the reaction of each individual. Several pre-operative visits may be necessary in order to give all the necessary information and avoid 'overloading' a bemused patient. Some patients may refuse to take in any information, and when this occurs medical and nursing staff should be kept informed.

Murrils (1983) suggests that pre-operative counselling should have four major aims:

1 To establish a relationship and provide support and reassurance for both the patient and spouse;
2 To elicit significant case history details and assess present communication skills;
3 To provide information regarding normal speech production;
4 To assist preparation for laryngectomy and subsequent voice loss, and to discuss alternative methods of alaryngeal communication.

The way in which the clinician handles the situation is crucial to the success of the pre-operative visit. This requires sensitivity in order to: (a) monitor the patient's responses to the information being given; and (b) adapt

*Figure 3 **Pre-operative evaluation***

Name _____ Unit no _____

Date of visit _____ Expected date of surgery _____

Evaluation carried out by _____

1 Check Medical Notes – date and extent of surgery _____
   _____

2 Basic Introduction – check information given and how much understood _____
   Mention altered breathing and aphonia _____
   _____

3 Oral/Physical Examination – check structure, function and mobility of:
   Lips _____
   Tongue _____
   Palate _____
   Jaw – upper and lower _____
   Neck _____
   Dentition _____
   Speech clarity, rate and accent _____
   _____

   Preferred language _____
   General communication _____
   Hearing acuity _____
   Is an aid worn? _____

4 Social and Family History _____
   _____

   Hobbies/interests _____
   _____

   Occupation _____
   Occupational speech needs _____
   _____

   Literacy _____

5 Laryngectomee Visitor requested _____
   Visitor arranged _____
   Video or audio tape _____

6 Spouse Counselling, including immediate post-operative appearance _____
   Spouse reaction and attitude to patient/surgery _____
   _____

7 Post-operative Communication – establish preferred means _____
   _____

8 General Information – stoma covers, change in senses, information leaflets ____
   _____

9 Date of Next Visit _____

10 Record Visit in Notes _____

the level of information accordingly. Anxiety and fear will lower the patient's capacity to receive and understand information.

Pre-operative Evaluation

Salmon (1986a) suggested a pre-operative evaluation sheet, and *Figure 3* is a modification of this which could be used. The following headings refer to the corresponding headings on the form.

I Check Medical Notes

The clinician needs to be fully aware of the patient's medical history. It is essential to ensure that it *is* a laryngectomy that is being planned and not a less or more extensive procedure. The patient should not be given unrealistic information; for example, someone about to undergo a pharyngo-laryngectomy would require different information from someone about to undergo a relatively straightforward laryngectomy.

The proposed date of surgery should be checked, along with the terminology used by the surgeon when explaining the proposed procedure, and the patient's reaction.

The amount and success of radiotherapy given should be noted – post-radiotherapy fibrosis may have adverse effects on rehabilitation, as can the need for post-operative radio- or chemotherapy, which may delay the commencement of therapy as the patient may not feel very well. However it should not be assumed that a patient who has received radiotherapy will automatically fail in voice acquisition.

Any general health problems which may affect general recovery, such as lung disease, mobility problems, hiatus hernia or other gastrointestinal problems, should be noted, as they may also affect the acquisition of oesophageal voice. Excess consumption of alcohol and tobacco will also affect recovery.

2 Basic Introduction

It is always wise to check that the patient *has* been seen by a member of the medical staff and told that they are to undergo a laryngectomy. This is usually quite easy to find out by asking whether they have seen the doctor that day, and what the doctor had to say. This will usually result in the clinician being told what the surgeon said. Where it is obvious that the patient has not understood (or does not wish to understand) what has been said, the clinician should report back to the medical staff and ask for the information to be given again.

It is also useful to know what other personnel have visited the patient, and what the patient's reaction was to their visits – ward staff are an invaluable source of such information.

During this initial visit, it is worth asking whether there are any aspects of the proposed procedures which the patient does not understand. It should be explained that the clinician is, as far as possible, prepared to answer any queries, and is able to refer on to another discipline if additional information is required.

Information given by the surgeon which should be reinforced by the clinician includes discussion of the permanent nature of the tracheostoma and the altered way of breathing this involves, and also reassurance that the patient will become accustomed to it in time.

It is also necessary to ensure that the patient is aware that there will be no voice at all post-operatively – many laryngectomees have stated that they believed they would be able to whisper. The realisation that they are totally voiceless is often a great shock to the best-prepared patient. The altered mechanisms for coughing and sneezing should be mentioned, although in some situations these will have been discussed by the physiotherapists during their visit.

The clinician can also familiarise the patient with certain post-operative features, such as the presence of a humidifier in the room, mentioning various drips and drainage tubes which may be in place, although it is obviously unwise to labour this point and end up with a terrified patient! (*See Chapter 2.*)

The fact that the operation itself is relatively painless, and that, once healing is complete, eating and drinking will be unaffected, is a positive feature which can be stressed. However the patient being prepared for extensive surgery needs slightly modified information.

3   Oral/Physical Examination

The structure and function of the oral musculature need to be compared pre- and post-operatively, and a thorough examination carried out. **Perry** (1983) suggests an excellent format for a pre- and post-operative oral examination, looking at:

▶ Lip and tongue structure, function and mobility, along with the efficiency of the lip seal and the range and strength of tongue tip elevation (the former being required for the bilabial injection method of air-charging and the latter for consonant injection of air). Damage to the hypoglossal nerve, resulting in tongue weakness, is a common complication of laryngectomy, and it is essential to be able to compare pre- and post-operative function, with therapy being planned around known physical limitations.

▶ The structure and movement of the hard and soft palate, as a certain amount of intra-oral pressure is required for oesophageal voice, especially when using consonant injection for air-charging. Excess nasality during pre-operative speech may be an indication of soft palate dysfunction, and this needs to be taken into consideration when working on intelligibility of speech post-operatively.

▶ Restricted jaw movements which can contribute to eating and drinking difficulties as well as unintelligibility of speech.

▶ The appearance of the neck, especially where there has been radiotherapy, since severe fibrosis or oedema will interfere with post-operative use of a neck-type artificial larynx, and an intra-oral aid will have to be considered instead.

▶ The condition of the patient's teeth or the presence and fit of dentures, as it is essential that dentures are well fitting before work on oesophageal voice is commenced. Likewise, decaying teeth are usually removed before surgery in order to reduce foci of infection post-operatively. Total absence of teeth or dentures will obviously affect articulation and therefore the ultimate clarity of speech, and must also be taken into consideration.

▶ The general rate and clarity of speech, along with the presence of strong regional or national accents, so that staff are prepared for the ease (or otherwise) of lip-reading post-operatively. Similarly, when the patient has a naturally loud voice, they should be prepared for reduction in volume associated with oesophageal voice, and females should be prepared for the lower pitch range.

▶ The patient's preferred language. If the clinician is not fluent in this language, it is important to establish a reliable means of communication, either by means of a common language, an interpreter or visual communication aids. It is so much easier for both clinician and patient to be able to establish some form of communication while the patient still has a voice, however poor.

▶ The patient's hearing acuity, and where a hearing aid has been prescribed, whether it is worn! Where there is an unresolved hearing problem, it is usual for the medical staff to deal with this, along with any dental problems.

The Northwestern Otolaryngology Communication Profile (**Logemann, Fisher and Becker**, 1980) can be used to assess the patient's communication in various situations, and can be used as a baseline for comparisons post-operatively.

4   Social and Family History

During conversation, the clinician should aim to discover information about the patient's family background, although some of this will be known from reading the medical notes. It is important to try to understand the social situation that they will be returning to, who the patient sees most often and relates to most effectively.

Discussion about interests, hobbies and, where appropriate, employment is useful, and realistic guidelines can be set for return to work. Where a person's occupation is dependent on speech, or where the working environment is dusty or noisy, return to work may be more difficult. The likelihood of the patient losing their job following surgery must also be kept in mind, as anxiety about this would contribute to increased tension during recovery. However it may be helpful to mention that there are laryngectomees in almost every profession.

The clinician should be aware of the patient's general reaction to this information, as well as the interaction between the patient and their family. Although difficulties in relationships may be purely a reaction to anxiety regarding the forthcoming surgery, it is well recognised that good family support is essential for complete rehabilitation of the laryngectomee.

Any financial difficulties which are mentioned should be referred, with the patient's permission, to the medical social worker, as well as queries regarding benefits or employment difficulties.

The clinician also needs to be aware of educational and literacy levels – it cannot be assumed that the patient will be able to communicate by writing post-operatively. This may be mentioned in relation to employment problems by the patient, or the spouse may mention it, although there is still a considerable stigma associated with poor literacy. Suggestions for coping with this are made in Section 7.

5   Laryngectomee Visitor

The clinician should offer to arrange a visit by a laryngectomee, or to show videos or play tapes of laryngectomee speakers, but the final decision on this should be the patient's. Some may prefer to wait until the post-operative period, feeling that they have enough to cope with until surgery is over. An initial reluctance may mask apprehension, and there is often a change of mind following a gentle enquiry. Both the patient's and the laryngectomee's spouses should be included wherever possible, but it is essential that the visitor is chosen with care.

Wherever possible, the visitor and patient should be matched for age and sex, and the visitor should be well adjusted and rehabilitated. They should be sociable and aware of the responsibilities of being an ambassador for the procedure!

The visit itself should be carefully managed by the clinician, arranging a suitable time and place for both visitor and patient. The visitor should be given basic information about the patient without any breach in confidentiality, and the patient told a little about the visitor. The clinician should accompany the visitor initially and make the introductions and initiate conversation if necessary, maintaining an awareness of how the visit is progressing.

If the patient is becoming distressed and obviously not recovering from this, then the visit should be curtailed. Where the visit is going well, it is possible for the clinician to leave first, with the visitor being 'primed' to assure the patient of a post-operative visit. This promise of continuity can be very reassuring for the patient.

Spouses often enjoy meeting in private, but it is essential that the visiting spouse is accurately informed about laryngectomy, and not prone to exaggeration! **Salmon** (1986a) in her study found that spouses appreciated the encouragement gained from others and the suggestions their visitors made about coping post-operatively.

6 Spouse Counselling

It is usual for the spouse to be well informed about laryngectomy by the surgeon pre-operatively, and for them to be fully aware of the implications.

The clinician's role is principally that of confirming the information already given, and it is especially useful to inform them about the appearance of their spouse immediately after the operation. In addition, the average length of time in theatre can be discussed, but with a reassurance that variations can and do occur, not necessarily because things are not going well.

Salmon (1986a) asked a large number of laryngectomees' spouses what information they felt would have been useful to have pre-operatively, and her results confirm the above approach. They wished to know about their partner's likely appearance post-operatively, and how to cope with the immediate physical and emotional needs. They also stated that the most difficult times had been when waiting during surgery, and the shock of the immediate post-operative appearance.

7 Post-operative Communication

This should be discussed with the patient and spouse and/or immediate family. It is important that, wherever possible, a functional means of communication is established pre-operatively. Most cope well with pen and paper, and in these cases the use of a 'Magic Slate', which can be 'written' on using a fingernail or any hard implement, prevents the frustration of never having a pen or blank paper available.

As mentioned earlier, it is not unusual to find that the patient's level of literacy is poor, making written communication difficult, if not impossible. Where this is known pre-operatively, arrangements can be made for a pictorial communication chart to be available. Commercially available charts can be used or individual ones devised, using loose-leaf sheets from photograph albums, which are conveniently covered with plastic. However illiteracy still carries a stigma, and this must be suspected if the laryngectomee is struggling with written communication post-operatively, or refusing to communicate at all.

20

8 General Information

The amount of information which can be assimilated pre-operatively by the patient is limited by anxiety about the procedure in many cases, but it may be relevant to give some general information.

Stoma care and covers can be mentioned briefly, along with change in smell and taste, laughing and coughing. Where and when therapy will commence is also useful for the patient to know, in addition to the reassurance that intelligible speech is possible post-operatively, and that there are a number of alternatives.

The mechanism of oesophageal voice can be outlined, as well as the use of electronic aids, and these should be introduced as an acceptable alternative, *not* as options after failure with oesophageal voice.

Where Surgical Voice Restoration is available, it can be mentioned as an option where patient selection requirements are met (*see Chapters 8 and 9*).

Written information leaflets, which contain more detailed information about certain aspects of being a laryngectomee, can be left with the patient (*see Useful Addresses*).

9 Date of Next Visit

The clinician should try to be specific as to when the next visit will be, so reinforcing a sense of continuity. Obviously all efforts should be made to keep this appointment, or the patient should be notified accordingly.

10 Record Visit in Notes

Medical and nursing staff need to be aware that the clinician's pre-operative visit has taken place, and to know of any relevant comments regarding the patient's attitude and reaction to the visit.

It can therefore be seen that, wherever possible, the basis for successful laryngectomee rehabilitation should be a structured, informative pre-operative visit, where both patient and clinician are given the opportunity to exchange and acquire information which will contribute towards the post-operative management of the laryngectomee.

Situations where a pre-operative visit is impossible or unavailable are dealt with in the next chapter.

CHAPTER 4
FIRST POST-
OPERATIVE VISIT

CHAPTER 4
FIRST POST-
OPERATIVE VISIT

Introduction

The first post-operative meeting between clinician and laryngectomee may occur in a number of different circumstances:

1   Immediately after surgery, where the clinician has met the laryngectomee pre-operatively;
2   Immediately after surgery, where the clinician has not visited the laryngectomee pre-operatively;
3   Some time after surgery, where the laryngectomee is ready to commence therapy.

Each of these situations will be discussed, and information which needs to be given at each stage outlined.

Where the Clinician Has Met the Laryngectomee Pre-operatively

This visit, which occurs very soon after surgery, usually the following day, is intended only for contact and reassurance that further visits will occur.

An effective means of communication will have been worked out pre-operatively, and it is wise to check that this is still effective, and that the laryngectomee is able to make needs known. Where it is apparent that the laryngectomee is failing with written means of communication, possibly owing to undisclosed literacy problems, an alternative means of communication, usually a pictorial communication chart, should be offered immediately.

Where the clinician is based 'on site', short daily visits to the laryngectomee can do much to establish rapport in preparation for later therapy. It is wise, however, to check medical notes for surgical and other reports, so that the laryngectomee is not given unrealistic goals. Points to note include:

▶ Extent and position of lesion. A tumour which has spread extensively or originated in locations other than the larynx itself, eg. post-cricoid region, will have resulted in more extensive surgery and an increased likelihood of recurrence.
▶ Other surgical procedures carried out. Where more extensive surgery has been necessary, therapy is likely to be more complex and recovery slower.

Where the pharyngeal area has been radically affected, or removed completely, acquisition of pseudo-voice will be affected.

▶ Radical neck dissection will affect the condition of the neck and placement of a neck-type artificial larynx, which should be used on the unaffected side. Where neck dissection has been bilateral, an intra-oral aid should be considered until healing is complete, when the situation can be reassessed. Neck dissection does not, however, necessarily prevent acquisition of oesophageal speech (**Hunt**, 1964).

▶ Surgery affecting the articulators, particularly the tongue. The tongue may be affected either by direct surgery, as in glossectomy or partial glossectomy, or indirectly by damage to its nerve supply. In such cases articulation will be affected, as well as the ability to inject air into the oesophagus to produce voice. The laryngectomee may be able to phonate using inhalation for air-charging (*see Chapter 5*) or by using an artificial larynx.

▶ Problems with healing, eg. unplanned fistulae. These will delay commencement of therapy, and can affect morale if not handled carefully. An intra-oral aid may be introduced to reduce frustration.

▶ Further treatment. Radiotherapy and chemotherapy may be planned post-operatively, and will also delay commencement of therapy; again an alternative means of communication needs to be established.

Where the Clinician Has Not Visited the Laryngectomee Pre-operatively

A number of factors may result in the laryngectomy being carried out without the clinician being able to carry out a pre-operative visit. The procedure may have been carried out as an emergency procedure; during the clinician's absence; or the surgeon may be unwilling for the visit to take place. (This attitude, although very difficult to comprehend, does, most unfortunately, still exist in some places!)

Where the clinician is visiting for the first time post-operatively, it is unwise to bombard the laryngectomee with too much information, when they are obviously still recovering, both physically and psychologically, after surgery. It is usually sufficient to introduce oneself and explain that you will be a regular visitor and will be involved with making their speech intelligible again. The spouse may be seen and a more detailed description of the speech clinician's role given (*see Chapter 10*).

Later, when the laryngectomee is more alert, the clinician can assess their general reaction to the surgery, and if necessary go through information which would have been given during the pre-operative visit. The details outlined in *Chapter 3* for the laryngectomee who is well prepared for surgery will naturally be required here as well. Even when a pre-operative visit has taken place, it is often necessary to reiterate some information, as before the operation the patient is often understandably preoccupied with the forthcoming surgery.

Salmon (1986a) reports on a study where laryngectomees listed information which they felt was most important to be given post-operatively. This included the reassurance that:
▶ they would learn to speak again by one method or another;
▶ there was a good chance for cure of the cancer following surgery;
▶ recovery was (or was not) progressing satisfactorily;
▶ they could be visited by a laryngectomee and spouse;
▶ an alternative voice could be produced;
▶ therapy would commence as soon as possible.

Other factors were related to cost and availability of therapy (the study was carried out in the United States), and requests for written self-care instructions. (*See Useful Addresses, 'Publications and Textbooks', for details of self-care leaflets.*)

The spouse's reaction to the surgery is also useful to note, as well as the laryngectomee's general attitude. Over-reliance on other people should be discouraged, as should over-protection by family members.

The pre-operative oral examination should be repeated, and any changes in physical structure or function noted. Where no pre-operative information is available, only a general assessment can be carried out, although any major problems may have been noted in the patient's medical notes (eg. dysarthria following a cerebrovascular incident).

As the laryngectomee recovers, and becomes keen to communicate, it is important that forced whispering is discouraged. In addition, the use of stoma blast (excessive noisy exhalation) as a substitute for voice should be stopped before it becomes established, and therefore very difficult to eradicate. Once the neck is healed, it may be advisable to start working with an artificial larynx where the laryngectomee is unable or unhappy to communicate by writing. The ENT surgeon should obviously be consulted before therapy commences.

Where the laryngectomee was visited pre-operatively, another visit by a laryngectomee may have been arranged, and this can be reassuring for the new laryngectomee. Where no visit occurred, similar guidelines to those outlined for the pre-operative visit by a laryngectomee should be followed (*see Chapter 3*).

Where the Laryngectomee is Ready to Commence Therapy

When the clinician's first contact with the laryngectomee is some time after surgery, slightly different information may need to be given.

In situations where the laryngectomee has been transferred to the clinician from another centre on discharge home, it is unusual for there to be many difficulties. In most cases, the laryngectomee will have been seen pre-operatively and/or post-operatively and the therapeutic process initiated. In these cases, the new clinician needs to check that all relevant information has been assimilated by the laryngectomee, who should be accompanied by the relevant transfer information, including the pre-operative evaluation.

The initial stage of establishing rapport and getting to know the patient may take a little longer, but, eventually, therapy should be able to proceed at a satisfactory pace. Where it is known that a different clinician will be responsible for a laryngectomee, it may be possible for the hospital clinician to arrange an introduction before the laryngectomee is discharged home.

There are more problems where the laryngectomee presents for therapy, seemingly 'out of the blue'. There may have been unexplained delays in referrals being sent, or a reluctance or inability to co-operate with therapy. Such delays should not be dwelled upon, but instead the clinician should work logically through a comprehensive assessment of the laryngectomee as they present. It may be necessary to reiterate much of the standard pre-operative information, suitably modified, and also to be prepared to correct faulty speech habits. These include stoma blast, forced whispering, and standing too close to people while talking to them – all of which develop in a short time when uncorrected, and can prove very difficult to eradicate once well established.

Spouse counselling in such situations will necessarily be more difficult, as they will already have had to cope with their altered situations, with a minimum of help. There may be a build-up of resistance to any help, or problems in accepting the situation.

It can be seen that the first post-operative visit, whenever it occurs, must be handled in the way most suitable for each individual, but must also be used as preparation for starting work on developing intelligible speech.

CHAPTER 5
OESOPHAGEAL VOICE

CHAPTER 5
OESOPHAGEAL VOICE

Introduction

The common assumption that laryngectomees speak by 'swallowing' air has been disproved, as a swallow is made up of different physiological features to those involved in air intake for oesophageal voice. (One of the more obvious differences is the absence of the peristaltic waves which occur during a swallow, moving the bolus of food towards the stomach; see **Diedrich and Youngstrom, 1977.**) **Salmon** (1986b) emphasises the necessity of establishing the difference between air intake and swallowing in the laryngectomee's mind – especially once some oesophageal voice has begun to emerge.

What is Oesophageal Voice?

There are many detailed descriptions of oesophageal voice, but, simply stated, it is the sound produced by a moving column of air in the oesophagus passing the pharyngo-oesophageal segment (P–E segment); as opposed to laryngeal voice, produced by a moving column of air from the lungs passing the vocal folds within the larynx.

(The term 'oesophageal voice' is used here as a specific term for sound produced in the oesophagus, whilst the term 'pseudo-voice' is used as a more general term, encompassing any alternative to laryngeal phonation, eg. pharyngeal or buccal voice.)

The air supply for oesophageal voice is usually taken in by a combination of one or more techniques: by using voiceless plosives to introduce air into the oesophagus (consonant injection); the action of the tongue against the palate (standard injection or glossopharyngeal press); or making use of the change in pressure around the oesophagus as air is taken into the lungs via the tracheostoma (inhalation).

If the P–E segment is relaxed, air can pass into the upper part of the oesophagus; the P–E segment then becomes the vibratory source for oesophageal voice. **Edels** (1983) and **Keith and Darley** (1986) contain more detailed and technical definitions of oesophageal voice.

How to Achieve Oesophageal Voice

Much has been written about techniques of teaching the acquisition of oesophageal voice, both from the clinician's and the laryngectomee's viewpoints. Over the years, there have been numerous suggested 'regimes' of exercises purporting to provide the 'ideal' programme to follow. The acquisition of oesophageal voice has been surrounded with a certain 'mystique', and it is therefore hardly surprising that inexperienced clinicians are often reluctant to take on this client group.

It may be helpful to quote here the wise words written by **Edels** (1983) that 'there is no one right way to obtain pseudo-voice' and that a 'flexible, eclectic approach which accommodates both the clinician and patient' is best. It is so often the way in which the clinician handles the laryngectomees, coping with their fears and anxieties and approaching therapy in a logical but flexible manner, which contributes to the success or otherwise of therapy.

The exercises suggested here for acquiring oesophageal voice are derived from many sources and from experience of working with laryngectomees who have achieved varying degrees of success. All who have worked with this client group will relate their failures, as well as successes – as yet, there is no absolutely guaranteed method for success!

When to Start

Work on developing oesophageal voice can commence once the ENT surgeon is happy that the oesophagus and surrounding structures are sufficiently healed for the nasogastric tube to be removed, and when normal feeding has been established for two or three days. This is usually at around ten days after surgery, although this can vary from person to person.

Medical consent must be obtained before commencing therapy, as developing oesophageal voice involves using muscles and other structures which have been operated on. Psychologically, however, it is essential for this to occur as soon as possible after surgery (**Bagshaw**, 1967; **Greene and Mathieson**, 1989). An unnecessary delay in starting therapy can impede later progress and motivation for therapy. Where therapy is delayed by surgical, medical or other complications, the clinician must be prepared to support the patient in other ways, such as ensuring an effective means of communication.

At each stage the laryngectomee should be given work to practise outside the therapy session – short but frequent practising is preferable to prolonged sessions, when fatigue and frustration reduce the likelihood of success. Five minutes' practice every waking hour can be suggested as a routine.

Wherever possible, the laryngectomee should be seen daily for therapy, with sufficient time being allocated for as long a session as is necessary. Where daily therapy is impossible, appointments should be arranged as regularly as possible. In situations where travelling difficulties would make daily attendance impracticable, it may be possible to delay the patient's discharge home for a short period, so that they are seen daily on the ward, for the initial period of therapy.

The First Therapy Session

The first therapy session needs to be handled carefully. Unnecessary stress and anxiety should be avoided. It is only natural that anticipation, apprehension and post-surgical discomfort may result in the laryngectomee becoming tense. Therefore, following a general introduction, it is often necessary to work on establishing a more relaxed posture and attitude.

Simple breathing work, aimed at establishing gentle rhythmic diaphragmatic movements, can also be beneficial, both in contributing to a more relaxed state and also in moving the focus of attention away from the head and neck area. Simple breathing exercises may be found in many standard texts on working with voice disorders (*see Bibliography*) or relaxation and yoga manuals.

The First Sound — Development Stages

Achieving the first oesophageal sound (physical constraints excepted) should be the aim of the first therapy session, but again, the clinician's attitude and approach can contribute much to the success or failure.

The following stages may be useful to work through in aiming to develop oesophageal voice.

Stage 1

Where the clinician is able to produce some oesophageal voice, it is useful to start by saying "Can you do this . . .?" and producing oesophageal voice for an open vowel /a/. At this stage it is unwise to attach undue importance to this sound, as this may increase the pressure on the patient to succeed and impede what may otherwise be naturally produced oesophageal voice. Often the patient will be able to copy this without knowing exactly what they are doing. If so, the first hurdle has been overcome.

Stage 2

Another approach is to ask whether they have had sound 'coming up' following meals, and whether they can make the same sound voluntarily. Although a belch is not the same as oesophageal voice, the sensation of air moving in the oesophagus is similar. Likewise, many small boys are, unknowingly, experts at producing oesophageal voice, and often, even as adults, they can remember what they used to do to produce a voluntary 'belch'. Natural resistance to 'belching' openly can be overcome by making the approach light-hearted, especially with the female laryngectomee. Often the initial sound produced will be relatively crude and the laryngectomee should be reassured that the sound quality will become refined with practice.

Stage 3

Any sound produced in this way should be praised, and followed by a request to do the same again. Where the sound is completely accidental, and voluntary repetition is impossible, then it is wise to go on to another activity, but emphasising that, having produced one sound, 'we know you can make it, now we just need to get it under control'.

If voicing is produced easily and repeatedly, go on to stage 5. Any method which enables the patient to achieve an acceptable, consistent voice should be reinforced and developed without undue concern about the precise method used.

Stage 4

Where sound is produced inconsistently, or not at all, it is important to continue working without making the patient feel that they have failed in any way. The importance of producing clearly articulated speech should be discussed, with explanation that certain sounds can contribute to intelligibility of speech if they are produced clearly. The clinician should demonstrate clearly and strongly articulated voiceless plosives, sibilants, affricates and blends of these: /p,t,k,s,ʃ,tʃ,sp,st,sk/. (It is also useful to produce whole words using these sounds, eg. 'spot', 'potato', 'sixty-six', 'scotch', demonstrating how much clearer they become when the voiceless sounds are produced with emphasis.) Using specific consonants to trigger voicing is known as consonant injection.

Single sounds or blends of voiceless plosives should be practised by the patient. Often their first attempts will result in weak sounds accompanied by excessive stoma blast (noisy, forceful exhalation of lung air from the stoma) as they continue to associate volume with increased breathing effort. Any stoma blast should be discouraged, with an explanation that this may affect the intelligibility and acceptability of their speech (**Shipp**, 1967). This also applies to excessive tension of the lips or tongue, which can be associated with excess tension in the P–E segment, and lessen the chances of phonation.

The sounds should be repeated in strings, but with each sound being produced as clearly as the first – often articulation becomes weaker as the repetitions increase, and this can lessen the chances of achieving voice, especially if repetition is too rapid. Twenty repetitions of each sound should be asked for, and the repetitions should be effortless and breathing quiet throughout.

Stage 5

Time spent on producing clearly articulated speech is never wasted, and it is essential that both patient and clinician feel relaxed and comfortable doing this, even if oesophageal voice has been produced easily and repeatedly in Stage 1. So often, inexperienced clinicians, pressurised by an understandably anxious patient, feel the necessity to 'go on to words' much too quickly.

When strings of voiceless plosives are produced well, the increased intra-oral pressure often results in some air being introduced into the oesophagus; this then results in oesophageal voice being produced easily and without forcing. The sound usually comes out as an /ʌ/ sound following the plosives, and, when this happens, the patient should be praised, while being told not to force the sound out, but to continue to concentrate on making the sounds clearly and without forcing from the stoma. Where sound is being produced consistently, it is important to discourage double pumping, where the articulatory movements are carried out twice if there is no sensation of air in the oesophagus. This, along with any other body movements or facial grimaces, can detract from speech and, once established, be difficult to eradicate.

Strings of voiceless phonemes can then be produced, with the patient being encouraged to produce a vowel after each one, /tatatatatatata/, /kakakakakakaka/ etc, without excess forcing. Where voicing is produced at first and then vanishes, it may be because strength of articulation has decreased, or because of excess tension in the oesophagus, specifically the P–E segment. This may be due to a build-up of tension during the session, or a hypertonic P–E segment. Suggestions for dealing with this will be found in the next chapter.

Stage 6

Alternatively, when attempting standard injection the clinician can get the laryngectomee accustomed to moving air around in the mouth, initially by blowing out the cheeks, and then by moving the air around, making a succession of sounds which involve compressing the air in the oral cavity using the tongue – not necessarily speech sounds!

Once the sensation of compressing air has been achieved, the laryngectomee can be encouraged to move the air back into the oesophagus by moving the tongue up against the hard palate. **Diedrich and Youngstrom** (1977) suggest that the patient imagines a bubble of air in the mouth, and squeezing it back into the oesophagus using the tongue. **Edels** (1983) suggests demonstrating the pumping action of the tongue against the hard palate, using one hand to represent the roof of the mouth, and the other, the tongue (glossopharyngeal press).

Again, where the clinician is able to demonstrate, the laryngectomee can gain feedback from watching and listening to the clinician, and feeling the effect of the air moving into the oesophagus by placing fingers gently on the clinician's neck, and listening to the 'klunk' as the oesophagus fills with air. This 'klunking' sound is associated with this method of air charging, and usually occurs because the patient is attempting to force too much air into the oesophagus. It can be used as a demonstration aid at this initial stage, but should be discouraged if it occurs in the patient's voicing attempts, by encouraging more relaxed efforts at injection.

When the patient has attempted to inject air into the oesophagus, they should be encouraged to bring the air back immediately to an /a/ sound – delay can result in any trapped air moving into the stomach of an inexperienced laryngectomee. The patient should attempt this a few times and then rest, whether voicing is successful or not, as it is likely that a certain amount of air has been swallowed, and will eventually be brought up from the stomach as a belch. They should be told to expect this, and, if it occurs, not to suppress the sound, but try to shape it into a vowel sound.

The laryngectomee may also complain of dryness in the mouth, and this is to be expected, both from increased articulatory movements and as a side-effect of anxiety. Alternatively, if the P–E segment is excessively tight, either as a result of surgery or of increased tension, continuous attempts at forcing air past it can result in the laryngectomee feeling very uncomfortable.

Stage 7

The inhalation method of air intake can be encouraged by getting the patient to open their mouth with the tongue lying flat. If they then take in a quick breath, the change in pressure around the oesophagus as the lungs expand can result in air being drawn into the oesophagus, in which case they will hear a 'click' as the air passes the P–E segment. The air should be brought back up to an /a/ sound, timed to coincide with expiration of lung air. Again there should be no forcing from the stoma.

The above techniques may be used exclusively or in combination by the patient.

Stage 8

When the patient has consistent and repeated experience of air moving in the oesophagus, it is useful to encourage them to describe what it feels like, in an attempt to increase kinaesthetic as well as auditory feedback for oesophageal sound. It is also essential that they can discriminate between oesophageal sound and that produced in the pharyngeal area.

The latter is usually due to excessive tension, resulting in the P–E segment becoming too tight, and sound being produced by air in the pharynx and the movements of the tongue against the pharyngeal wall. The sound produced is typically high in pitch and short in duration. Pharyngeal voice may be produced at times when the laryngectomee is experimenting with producing sound, and the clinician should increase the patient's auditory awareness, contrasting the pharyngeal with the lower-pitched oesophageal voice. General relaxation, and asking for a lower-pitched sound, should help reduce its occurrence in most cases.

Words should not be attempted until repeated strings of sounds can be produced with voicing 90 per cent of the time. Breathing throughout should be quiet and speech attempts unimpeded by facial grimaces or unnecessary movements. If these are curtailed as they emerge, much work can be avoided later.

Stage 9

The first words to be attempted should be chosen carefully, and be full of sounds which facilitate phonation. Those laryngectomees using inhalation or standard injection will prefer words with voiced phonemes or vowels at the beginning (for examples, see List 1 at the end of the chapter). Those using consonant injection prefer words beginning with voiceless sounds (List 2).

Stage 10

Two-syllable utterances and two-word combinations can then be attempted (List 3).

Stage 11

By this time oesophageal voice may be emerging during speech attempts unconnected with exercises, but the patient should be discouraged from deliberate attempts to use the new voice for conversation at this stage. It is unlikely that control is such that oesophageal voice can be used for connected speech without resultant forcing or developing bad habits. Where oesophageal voice occurs automatically, this should be accepted as an 'added bonus' at this stage.

Stage 12

Two-word utterances should be followed by phrases of increasing length and complexity, and, at this stage, all speech sounds can be used. Patients should be reminded to check that they have sufficient air in the oesophagus at all times – since only about 15 ml of air is available per charge, it is essential that the best use is made of this air. Articulating in a slow, relaxed manner will help, as will reminders to 'top-up' or re-charge during pauses in speech.

Stage 13

Replenishment of air, or 'topping-up' should be practised so that it becomes natural and rapid. Here again, the awareness of what is happening during oesophageal voice production (see Stage 8) is invaluable for both patient and clinician. The time lapse between attempts to charge the oesophagus and voice production is known as the latency period, and in fluent speech 'this latency period needs to be in the region of 0.5s' (**Edels**, 1983).

Stage 14

Names of family members, greetings and everyday phrases should be practised as preparation for using oesophageal voice in connected speech. (A useful therapeutic tool is a prepared list of phrases and sentences of increasing length, which allows the clinician to spend valuable therapy time working directly with the patient, not trying to think up sentences!)

Stage 15

Some phonemes may prove more difficult than others for the laryngectomee to produce – typically, those using consonant injection prefer voiceless sounds, whereas those using inhalation and standard injection for air-charging prefer words beginning with vowels or voiced consonants. Where these are identified, time should be spent on mastering difficult sounds in isolation and in words. By this stage, oesophageal voice should be being produced at will, with the patient being able to concentrate on mastering difficult sounds.

For example, the nasal sounds, /m,n,ŋ/ can be worked on by prolonging a vowel and closing the lips halfway through, or producing strings of /amama-mamam/ sounds, then working towards producing /aaamm/ and finally /m/ on its own. The sound /n/ can be worked on in the same way, but usually, once one nasal sound has been mastered, the others are assimilated easily into speech.

Stage 16

Connected speech and reading passages can then be worked on, along with work on phrasing and timing. An efficient oesophageal speaker can expect to produce eight to ten syllables on one intake of air, and therefore, during connected speech, the laryngectomee needs to be able to 'top up' the air. This should be practised along with pausing at suitable points during connected speech. Laryngectomees should be reassured that pausing is an acceptable part of everyone's speech. Rushing, and 'gulping' for air, should be discouraged, as they distract from speech as well as being inefficient methods of air intake.

Stage 17

When the laryngectomee makes the first attempt at using oesophageal speech in conversation outside the therapy session, failure to phonate should not be seen as a complete disaster – often, under stress, they forget all they have learnt, and panic. It is therefore advisable for the clinician to work on using oesophageal voice in different situations with the patient and also to accompany them on non-threatening speech assignments. Hospital outpatients' coffee bars are invaluable for this!

Assessment

Periodic assessment of the laryngectomee is essential throughout therapy, for monitoring progress and planning the next stages. **Perry** (1983) mentions the 'halo effect', with clinicians presuming that 'a laryngectomee must have improved because he has been attending therapy regularly', and this is far more likely to occur where the clinician has had limited exposure to laryngectomees and the varying standards of oesophageal speakers.

There are various means of assessing the laryngectomee, both informally and formally, and, using these, it is much easier to be objective and to plan therapy accordingly. **Berlin** (1963) outlines four measures of skill in an efficient oesophageal speaker, who would be able to:

(a) Phonate virtually 100 per cent of the time, on demand, after 10–14 days of therapy;

(b) Achieve a latency of 0.2 to 0.6 seconds between inflation and phonation by the eighteenth day of therapy;

(c) Sustain /a/ for between 2.2 and 3.6. seconds by the twenty-fourth day of therapy;

(d) Phonate 8–10 plosive syllables per overt inflation by the twenty-fifth day of therapy.

It is often difficult to be objective when assessing our own patients, and therefore useful to be aware of formal assessments, which can be used with laryngectomees. These include:

▶ Oesophageal Voice Assessment (**Gardner**, 1971);
▶ Alaryngeal Speech Checklist (**Berry**, 1976) which can be used with artificial larynx users as well;
▶ Wepman Scale of Speech Proficiency (**Wepman *et al.***, 1953);
▶ Hyman Rating Scale (**Hyman**, 1957);
▶ Northwestern Otolaryngology Communication Profile (**Logemann, Fisher and Becker**, 1980) which is given pre- and post-operatively.

Where formal assessments are unavailable, the following guidelines may be useful for assessing oesophageal communication, and for improving performance. **Keith and Darley** (1986) suggest that quality, fluency and clarity should be monitored.

1   Quality of oesophageal voice can be improved by:

(a)   Control of stoma air – reducing force of expiration and providing visual and auditory feedback about stoma blast. (This can be done by using a tissue placed in front of the stoma, or placing an amplifier microphone directly in front of the stoma, which will amplify the stoma blast.)
(b)   Reduction of any sound produced when trapping air by taking in less air, and with less force.
(c)   Getting rid of facial and body movements associated with speech attempts.
(d)   Reducing consonant distortion of vowels – especially when using consonant injection for air intake. This can be reduced by auditory training and practising silent intake.
(e)   Developing inflection. The fundamental frequency of oesophageal voice in an average male is about 65 Hz, half that of a laryngeal speaker. Pitch range is often reduced to 5–8 tones. Intonation patterns can be practised using vowels and short phrases, aiming for maximum use of the available range.
(f)   Developing proper rhythm – working on stressing appropriate words, using available pitch and volume changes.
(g)   Developing sufficient loudness – oesophageal voice is less intense than laryngeal voice. Average oesophageal voice intensity is 40–50 dB, with an approximate range of only 20 dB. (Laryngeal voice has an average intensity of 65–70 dB with a range up to 95 dB.) Digital pressure on the neck at the level of the P–E segment may help to increase volume, as may turning the head slightly to one side, or wearing a pressure band.

2   Fluency of oesophageal voice production is achieved by:

(a)   Consistency of production. The aim is for quick intake of air and long duration, as in laryngeal voice. Consistency is based on success in phonating per number of attempts and, as previously noted, 90 per cent success should be the rate aimed at. Latency during air intake needs to be less than 1 second, and this can be worked on by attempting repeated phonation at regular intervals, eg. every fourth beat, and gradually shortening the period between attempts.
(b)   Increasing duration of phonation. Initially, oesophageal phonation may last less than 1 second, whereas 2–3 seconds should be aimed at, by

working on reducing volume of phonation (so that available air lasts longer), working on producing increasing lists of vowels, and relaxed, controlled intake of air.

(c)   Working on increasing the number of words per air charge, by encouraging relaxed intake of air and slow controlled expiration; working on gradually increasing phrases and groups of words, eg. 'check', 'check it', 'check it out'.

(d)   Making sure word groupings follow each other without noticeable pause – that is, by working on quiet and efficient air intake and use of available air.

(e)   Improving overall rate of speech without losing quality – a good oesophageal speaker can achieve rates of between 80 and 110 words per minute (normal prose reading in a laryngeal speaker is 150–165 wpm).

3   Clarity of oesophageal speech can be achieved by:

(a)   Making sure articulation of each sound is accurate; for example, patients who use inhalation and standard injection methods of air intake tend to make voiceless phonemes voiced, and those using consonant injection may tend to distort vowel sounds at the beginning of words. Voiced phonemes can be made to sound more intelligible by prolonging vowels, voiceless sounds more intelligible by shortening vowels.

(b)   Checking articulation in words by working on contrasting word pairs (see List 4) alone and in phrases.

(c)   Checking articulation in connected speech.

Not all laryngectomees can learn to use oesophageal voice, but those that do should receive therapy planned to enable them to achieve their potential. Continuous assessment, and working on refining the voice produced, can contribute towards this.

Word Lists

List 1

at	it	each	odd	up	on
am	in	eat	or	our	off
eye	ice	aim	oat	add	if
bat	back	bark	bad	bored	beard
bear	bard	been	bath	both	bed
dot	dog	dig	date	dote	debt
dark	din	dud	dear	do	day
go	get	gate	gale	gap	gun
gain	gull	goes	gas	girl	gape

List 2

par	pour	poor	pay	pea	purr
pat	pot	pit	pack	peat	port
tar	tea	tie	two	tap	toe
top	tip	tick	tock	tape	tight
car	key	core	care	cat	cap
cup	cut	cape	kit	kite	catch
chop	chip	shop	ship	fish	fit
spot	sport	scot	skate	stop	step

List 3

apple	over	under
eat it	each one	add it
on each	aim it	off on
I am	you are	is it
bat it	bad back	get it
dear girl	big bed	gas bill
pocket	ticket	chatter
tip top	kit kat	tick tock
take care	put it	push it
pour out	patch it	tea pot

List 4

pie/buy	to/do	pour/bore
tea/D	pear/bear	cap/gap
cut/gut	cape/gape	tip/dip
chin/gin	fan/van	are/tar
cut/cup	chain/Jane	jeep/cheap

CHAPTER 6
DIFFICULTIES IN ACQUISITION

aged initially. Similarly, a delay in switching on results in initial voiced sounds being difficult to comprehend or being perceived as voiceless. Early reminders to 'switch on' only when speech movements are initiated should ensure improved timing, as should encouragement to slow down the rate of speech initially, so that there is time to remember to 'switch on'.

5. Articulation

CHAPTER 6
DIFFICULTIES IN ACQUISITION

Introduction

Not all laryngectomees will achieve functionally useful oesophageal voice, and the proportion who are quoted as failing to develop voice varies from source to source, from 43 per cent (**King *et al.*,** 1968) to 98 per cent (**Hunt,** 1964). The clinician working with laryngectomees needs to be aware of the problems which may affect voice acquisition, and **Duguay** (1979) puts these into four categories:

1. Anatomical and physiological reasons;
2. Psychological and sociological reasons;
3. Teaching and learning reasons;
4. Only God knows – a term for a small proportion of laryngectomees who fail to acquire voice and where the reasons for failure cannot be determined. A more detailed description of these categories follows.

Anatomical and Physiological Reasons

The acquisition of oesophageal voice may be hindered by general medical problems, present pre-operatively or resulting from the surgical or therapeutic procedures. Specific difficulties are listed by **Duguay** (1979) under four stages of voice production, a disruption in one or more of which may result in difficulty in acquisition of oesophageal voice:

Stage I   – inability to force air into the oesophagus;
Stage II – inability to retain air in the oesophagus;
Stage III – inability to return air from the oesophagus; and
Stage IV – problems with the pharyngo-oesophageal sphincter (P–E segment).

Stage I   Inability to Force Air into the Oesophagus

The production of oesophageal voice is dependent on the introduction of a certain amount of air into the oesophagus. Anatomical and physiological reasons for not achieving this may include:

(a)   Cranial nerve damage: radical neck dissection may result in disruption of oral sensations and restricted tongue movement. This may make the injection method of air-charging more difficult or impossible in some cases. Careful examination of the oral structure and function pre- and post-operatively, as well as detailed information of the surgical procedures carried out, may alert the clinician to the likelihood of this problem. The use of the inhalation method of air intake may be more appropriate in these cases.

(b) Velopharyngeal incompetency: structural problems such as a cleft palate, bifid uvula, congenitally short palate or neurological palatal insufficiency may contribute to difficulty in introducing air into the oesophagus, as it is necessary to close off the nasopharynx in order to build up intra-oral pressure.

(c) High pouches above the level of the P–E segment: these may result in increased pressure being necessary to introduce air into the oesophagus. **Simpson** *et al.* (1972) described these pouches, which may trap air, mucus and saliva, and affect the voice quality. Videofluoroscopic studies designed to study the structure of the tract during attempts at voicing may reveal the presence of such pouches, which must be taken into consideration when a laryngectomee is experiencing difficulties with voice acquisition.

(d) Inability to relax the P–E segment voluntarily: this would make introduction of air into the oesophagus more difficult. Where the P–E segment is resistant to opening, either structurally or as a result of psychological tension (**Faulkener**, 1940; **Greene**, 1947), the air remains in the area above the P–E segment, resulting in a neoglottis situated at the base of the tongue. Sound produced is typically high-pitched, constricted in quality and limited in duration. **Duguay** (1979) suggests that, in teaching relaxation and anxiety reduction, especially in relation to speech attempts, the clinician may be able to contribute to the relaxation of this sphincter. In severe cases, pharyngo-oesophageal dilation by bouginage or surgical myotomy may be considered.

(e) A too flaccid P–E segment: as a result, the neoglottis is poorly defined, and therefore air intake is inefficient. (This difficulty will be discussed in more detail later.)

Stage II   Inability to Retain Air in the Oesophagus

and

Stage III   Inability to Return Air from the Oesophagus

When air has been introduced into the oesophagus, it is necessary for it to be retained briefly in the oesophagus before being returned into the oropharynx.

(a) An incompetent cardiac (distal) sphincter, which separates the oesophagus from the stomach, is a feature of hiatus hernia. **Wolfe** *et al.* (1971) showed evidence of a number of 'failed' oesophageal speakers who complained of symptoms consistent with the presence of a hiatus hernia – heartburn, regurgitation (reflux), chest pain and food 'sticking' in the throat. Following attempts at air-charging, laryngectomees with cardiac sphincter insufficiency will typically complain of a substantial amount of air in the stomach and a feeling of distension and discomfort at every attempt to introduce air into the oesophagus. A competent cardiac sphincter seems to be necessary for successful retention of air in the oesophagus. Attempts to produce oesophageal voice may exacerbate the symptoms of a hiatus hernia, and in these cases the temporary use of an artificial larynx is recommended until the hernia is surgically treated. Where surgery is not an option, permanent use of an artificial larynx should be considered.

(b) Achalasia is a disorder of the lower oesophageal area: lack of lower oesophageal relaxation results in the food bolus being obstructed during swallowing. This has serious implications for general well-being as well as voice acquisition. It is a progressively deteriorating condition which has to be treated surgically, but even then complete restoration of bolus motility is not achieved, owing to neurological changes which cannot be reversed.

Stage IV Problems with the Pharyngo-oesophageal (P–E) Sphincter

The P–E segment is composed of the cricopharyngeal muscle and fibres from the inferior pharyngeal constrictor muscle and upper oesophagus, and is generally shown to be located between C5 and C6 (**Diedrich and Young-strom**, 1966).

Problems with the P–E segment can result in inability to introduce air into the oesophagus, retain it or recover the air. **Perry and Edels** (1985) emphasise the importance of the tonicity of the P–E segment, and outline an objective evaluation procedure for investigating the tonicity of the sphincter, involving videofluoroscopy during three separate procedures:

(a) Barium swallow,
(b) Attempted phonation,
(c) Air insufflation test (**Taub and Bugner**, 1973).

Laryngectomees were categorised as 'good' or 'failed' oesophageal speakers. Good oesophageal speakers were those with a tonic P–E segment, who showed on (a) an open oesophagus, with fast motility of the bolus; on (b) one visible P–E segment, and there was good voice with a good oesophageal air reservoir; and on (c) good voice. In their study Perry and Edels categorised 'failed' oesophageal speakers along a continuum of P–E segment tonicity, which included the following features.

(i) *Hypotonic segment* The barium swallow showed good dilation of the oesophagus, with fast motility of the bolus, but on attempted phonation no P–E segment was visible. On air insufflation a whispery/weak voice was heard, or no phonation at all. This may be remedied by applying digital pressure to the neck after air intake but prior to phonation, resulting in improved adduction of the oesophageal mucosa and the formation of a temporary P–E segment. The use of a pressure band to increase resistance anteriorly to the flaccid P–E segment may also be beneficial (**Duguay**, 1979) or changing head position, turning gently to one side to improve voice quality.

(ii) *Hypertonic segment* The barium swallow showed slight narrowing of the tract but with some dilation. During attempted phonation one tight or two P–E segments were visible, with resultant poor voice, often in bursts of sound as the segment was incapable of releasing air smoothly. During insufflation a better voice was achieved on gentle air-blowing.

(iii) *Spasm* The hypertonicity of the segment was severe; on barium swallow there was slight narrowing of the tract, but on attempted phonation a very tight segment was visible, with very poor or no voice. Significantly, on insufflation there was still no voice, and the very tight P–E segment was only able to release air explosively. The insufflation test was the most useful in distinguishing between the mild hypertonic segment and spasm. In cases of hypertonicity, **Singer and Blom** (1981) suggest pharyngo-oesophageal myotomy to release the excess muscle tonicity. **Perry and Edels** (1985) report that, following myotomy, the laryngectomees were able to acquire oesophageal voice, with therapy aimed at teaching inhalation as a method of air intake.

(iv) *Stricture* During barium swallow there was little or no dilation, dysphagia was reported, and there was slow motility of the bolus. On attempted phonation little or no air reached the oesophagus, and there was no voice. On insufflation the oesophagus inflated, but there was no voice as the P–E segment did not open to allow the passage of air back into the oropharynx. **Singer and Blom** (1981) suggest that this may be repaired by using a two-stage pharyngectomy and flap repair for surgical removal of the stricture.

Apart from the specific features mentioned above, other anatomical and physiological factors may contribute to problems in voice acquisition.

Healing impeded by unplanned fistulae

In all cases, commencement of oesophageal voice training is delayed until the vocal tract and surrounding tissues are healed to an acceptable level, but, where there are severe or recurring fistulae, further surgery may be necessary to encourage healing. The laryngectomee should be supplied with an effective alternative means of communication, usually an artificial larynx. An intra-oral aid can be used without exerting pressure on the healing neck tissues, or alternatively a neck-type aid can be used against the cheek.

Hearing loss in either the laryngectomee or spouse

This may affect the successful acquisition of voice. Self-monitoring, which is an important feature of successful voice acquisition, is affected if the laryngectomee is hard of hearing. Where a hearing-aid has been prescribed, it is wise to check that it is in good working order, and being worn. Stoma blast must be monitored by tactile feedback by placing a hand in front of the stoma, or by amplifying the stoma blast using a microphone.

Where the laryngectomee's spouse is hard of hearing, straining and forcing to make themselves heard by their spouse may result in the laryngectomee acquiring bad habits during speech attempts, typically stoma blast. Amplification at an early stage of speech rehabilitation may be useful, as well as suggestions for making communication as effective as possible, maintaining face-to-face contact, and reducing extraneous distracting noises.

General ill-health

This may affect the laryngectomee's ability to concentrate and motivation for therapy. Chronic chest diseases often occur alongside laryngeal malignancy, and the laryngectomee may have to cope with persistent coughing along with copious production of mucus. Damage to the thyroid gland during surgery may result in hormone imbalance, necessitating medical intervention to restore the hormonal balance and general well-being of the patient.

Lack of co-ordination in diaphragmatic movements

This may result in problems co-ordinating diaphragmatic movements with those of the neoglottis. In their study, **Samuel and Adams** (1976) concluded that the neoglottis relaxes as the diaphragm descends, and subsequently, in preparation for speech, the diaphragm begins to ascend. They also reported that no patient with poorly co-ordinated diaphragmatic movements had good voice.

Psychological and Sociological Reasons

Where there are no apparent anatomical or physiological reasons for difficulties in acquisition of oesophageal voice, other features which may affect success may be classed as psychological or sociological ones, in the laryngectomee and/or their family. These may include signs of depression, fear of recurrence of the disease, and low motivation.

Depression

It is usual, as with any loss, for the patient to go through some reactive depression, either post-diagnosis, immediately before surgery, or at some time later. Often, within the environment of the hospital, with all the facilities available, along with supportive, knowledgeable staff, the full realisation of life as a laryngectomee does not become apparent. Many laryngectomees react badly when they first return home; careful preparation, along with instruction for the carers, can help prepare all concerned for this occurrence. In addition, they should be helped, by a trained counsellor if necessary, to accept the reality of the loss, encouraged to experience the pain of grief, and therefore to adjust to the changed environment. They can also be encouraged to reinvest their emotional energy in tackling their new situation.

Where depression appears to be more severe, resulting in a fatigued, listless person, preoccupied with self, lacking interest in former activities and showing increased irritability, then the clinician should not hesitate to suggest referral to a more qualified professional, whether for prescription of a suitable anti-depressant drug or for therapy. Often the clinician, during regular therapeutic contacts, will be the professional most likely to notice, or to be told about, the depression by a concerned carer.

Fear of Recurrence of the Disease

This may be severe, resulting in anxiety and unwillingness to participate in therapy for fear of triggering further disease (**Salmon**, 1986d). Fear of death post-operatively may be foremost in their minds, blocking off all other thoughts. The clinician should ensure that the laryngectomee has an understanding of what has happened, and that their understanding is at an appropriate level. Medical details should be explained and reinforced by the surgeon or nursing staff, so that ignorance does not precipitate unnecessary fear, which can affect rehabilitation.

Dependency

A change in dependency may affect the patient's motivation. A person who is independent before surgery may become totally dependent after it. Although sight or dexterity problems may prevent the laryngectomee from being totally self-caring, they should be encouraged to resume as much of their previous independence as possible.

Motivation

Motivation was seen by **Stoll** (1958) as the most important factor in determining the success of voice acquisition. The individual's communication needs must be assessed and a programme devised accordingly. A laryngectomee who lives alone may have little need or desire to communicate, and may be less motivated to succeed than a more socially active person. However **Shanks** (1986b) states that, 'if the desire to talk is strong enough and if there is an opportunity to learn, he can learn by one means or another'.

Anxiety

Anxiety about new body functions, the altered method of breathing, smelling and tasting, may be severe. Patients may dislike the sound of oesophageal voice initially, and prefer to use an artificial larynx, or not to speak at all. Again, explanation of structure and function before and after surgery should ensure that the laryngectomee is aware of the altered body functions, and any initial dislike of oesophageal voice may be altered by introducing the new laryngectomee to a well-adjusted, competent oesophageal speaker. (A fuller discussion of this is to be found in *Chapter 3*. It is, however, always necessary to be realistic when comparing patients, and to assess each person's potential individually.)

Finance and Occupation

Financial and occupational worries may be overwhelming, making concentration for speech rehabilitation difficult. Where the laryngectomee is the 'bread-winner', financial problems may be exacerbated by threats of redundancy. Unfortunately, many laryngectomees face redundancy after the operation, especially where there is a strong verbal component to the work. Early introduction to an artificial larynx may ensure early return to work, and financial worries may be helped by referral to the social worker. In addition, it may be possible for the clinician to make contact with the employers via their personnel department, and, by informing them of post-operative employment possibilities, reduce ignorance and routine dismissal. If return to work is anticipated, this early contact may be useful for later planning for specific work situations.

Body Image

Female laryngectomees often experience problems adjusting to the altered body image, feelings of being unattractive, and dislike of oesophageal voice because of its relatively low pitch (**Greene and Mathieson**, 1989). A slight increase in pitch may be achieved by using digital pressure and experimenting with different head positions. Alternatively, they may choose to rely on an artificial larynx.

Salmon (1986a) describes specific social and personality factors related to good oesophageal voice. The criteria for successful acquisition of voice include age at operation, a high personal achievement level, favourable self-concept, good body image, less depression and low levels of anxiety.

Teaching and Learning Reasons

The laryngectomee may be unable or unwilling to acquire oesophageal voice or, unfortunately, the clinician may be a poor teacher! Factors affecting the laryngectomee's ability to learn include the following.

Low Intelligence

Where the laryngectomee is unable to grasp the technique of oesophageal voice production owing to low intelligence, **Perry** (1983) suggests that imitation may be successful, especially when used on an intensive, daily basis. It may be possible for the laryngectomee to be admitted for in-patient treatment where travelling distance causes problems.

Illiteracy

This problem may become apparent in the immediate post-operative period when the laryngectomee is unwilling or unable to communicate needs by writing. During this period a pictorial communication chart may be used, along with introduction to an artificial larynx as soon as possible. Where illiteracy exists in isolation, that is without accompanying low intelligence, it has been the author's experience that acquisition of oesophageal voice can be achieved by intensive therapy, reinforced by audio-tapes for home practice. Concern about 'exposing' their illiteracy may retard the patient's progress in the initial stages of therapy, and it is essential that the clinician manages this, not as an insurmountable social stigma but as an additional feature of the individual's situation.

Dementia/Senility

Senility and general mental deterioration as found in dementia are usually contraindications for successful acquisition of oesophageal voice, and often for successful use of an artificial larynx. These patients should be equipped with alternative means of communication, relevant to their individual needs.

Alcoholism

The high incidence of alcoholism among laryngectomees is well known, usually being a continuation of a pre-operative problem, not a result of surgery. The immediate post-operative recovery may be affected by symptoms of alcohol withdrawal, and behavioural problems may become evident during rehabilitation, with gross motor inco-ordination, slurred speech and disruptive behaviour. There may be impaired comprehension and execution of commands, along with non-compliance with therapeutic practice material. Attendance may be poor. In general, the clinician will require to involve other professionals where a laryngectomee is felt to be showing signs of alcoholism, as progress is usually poor where alcoholism is uncontrolled.

Teaching Difficulties

The fact that few clinicians experience regular contact with laryngectomees at varying stages of rehabilitation contributes to a proportion of laryngectomees failing to acquire oesophageal voice because we are poor teachers. Where a clinician has limited experience it is essential to become aware of how good an oesophageal speaker can be – many clinicians accept inferior levels of voice quality, believing that 'anything is better than nothing', and therefore leave their clients ill-equipped and disappointed in their achievements. Regular assessment of the laryngectomee in therapy may give a more objective format to planning.

Regular updating of information is essential when dealing with this client group, and many excellent courses are organised, enabling inexperienced and experienced clinicians to update their information. In the United Kingdom, the National Association of Laryngectomee Clubs runs several study days each year, for clinicians and often laryngectomees as well, and can be contacted for details of future events. In the United States, the Mayo Clinic Laryngectomee Rehabilitation Seminars and Voice Institutes have achieved international acclaim for their standard of tuition for professionals and laryngectomees alike. In other countries, clinicians are advised to contact their professional bodies or laryngectomee associations, for example the International Association of Laryngectomees (*see Useful Addresses*).

Lack of therapy provision by a clinician competent in dealing with laryngectomee rehabilitation may occur as a result of travelling constraints where a laryngectomee lives at a distance from the contact clinic. As mentioned previously, it may be possible to arrange hospital admission for intensive therapy, as well as home therapy by means of audio-tapes. Distance learning – preferably with the support of a local relative or carer, who can be suitably instructed by the clinician – must, however, be monitored closely as poor speech habits may develop more quickly where the laryngectomee is not supervised by a suitable trained professional.

Only God Knows

There will be a few individuals who fail to acquire voice, but do not appear to fall into any of the above categories. Where this occurs, the clinician, providing they have fully investigated all channels, should not devote critical treatment time attempting to uncover the causative factor, but rather concentrate on providing the laryngectomee with an alternative means of communication appropriate to their individual situation and needs.

CHAPTER 7
COMMUNICATION AIDS

CHAPTER 7
COMMUNICATION AIDS

Introduction

This chapter will discuss the use of communication aids with laryngectomees – specifically artificial or electronic larynges, whether and when they should be used – as well as a description of some of the most commonly available. Suggestions for therapy using communication aids are also included.

Why Use Communication Aids?

A percentage of laryngectomees will fail to acquire oesophageal speech; in the past, they were often only considered suitable for communication aids after this failure. **Salmon** (1986c) explored the myth (which, unfortunately, some professionals persist in believing) that the use of an artificial larynx in some way impedes acquisition of oesophageal voice, and found no research data to support this idea. Indeed, studies by **Gates *et al.*** (1982) and by Salmon herself showed that laryngectomees actually benefited from early experience of using an artificial larynx. Some of the benefits of early use of artificial larynges included the following.

Rapid Communication

The intra-oral type of electronic speech aid (eg. Cooper-Rand) can be used very soon after surgery, as the mouth-piece does not interfere with the surgically affected neck area.

The use of neck-type devices should be delayed until healing is well under way, as local discomfort and swelling may impede their effective use.

Less Frustration

The ability to communicate using speech at an early stage must contribute to reducing the effects of frustration during speech attempts. Emotional stress and the sense of isolation the patient feels at being unable to make oneself heard may be reduced.

Reduction of Bad Habits

Often, during the initial post-operative period, the new laryngectomee is tempted to use noisy expiration (stoma blast) as a substitute for voice. If not curtailed at an early stage, this can become a distracting feature of later speech attempts – reducing intelligibility by masking oesophageal voice and also reducing the acceptability of speech for listeners. The ability to produce audible speech using an artificial larynx can help reduce the possibility of this happening.

Occupational and Social Benefits

On discharge home, the use of an aid allows the laryngectomee to consider resuming previous social and work activities as soon as medically advisable – even when the occupation demands use of the voice.

Less Stress During Oesophageal Voice Training

Where the laryngectomee can already communicate audibly using an aid, the stress engendered by striving to succeed during attempts at producing oesophageal voice may be reduced. Increased tension in the head and neck area can only mitigate against attempts at oesophageal voice production. Tension can be intense when the laryngectomee is anxious to be able to produce audible, intelligible speech again. In addition, work on producing intelligible voiceless plosives and generally clear articulation when introducing the artificial larynx will always be useful in any subsequent work on oesophageal voice acquisition. Conversely, where a laryngectomee fails to acquire oesophageal voice, if the artificial larynx is already established as an acceptable means of communication, then the false assumption that they are only used by 'failures' is less likely to be made.

After Extensive Surgery

After extensive surgery, such as pharyngo-laryngo-oesophagectomy, where the likelihood of producing oesophageal voice is reduced, the early use of an aid can help restore effective communication at an earlier stage. This also applies in cases where the whole of the tumour cannot be removed and the prognosis for recovery is poor. In these cases, rapid, effective restoration of intelligible speech is a primary concern. Certain modifications during their use may be necessary (eg. placement of neck-type aids) and these will be discussed later in the chapter.

Types of Artificial Larynx Available

Attempts to produce an acceptable substitute for the removed larynx have been made since the very first laryngectomy was carried out by Bilroth in 1873, when his assistant, Gussenbauer, fashioned a silver prosthesis with a metallic reed. One end of the prosthesis was inserted into the tracheostoma, with the other end inserted into the pharynx. Expired air produced vibration of the reed and the sound produced was a substitute voice.

Since then, the development of (a) artificial larynges, and (b) voice prostheses has advanced substantially, and these now constitute two separate fields of voice rehabilitation. (Surgical voice restoration is discussed in the following chapters.)

There are basically two types of artificial larynx available – pneumatic and electronic. The former is powered by lung air and the latter by batteries. Electronic aids are divided into intra-oral and neck types. For those readers unfamiliar with communication aids, a brief description follows.

1   *The pneumatic artificial larynx* involves a cap which fits over the tracheostoma, shunting exhaled air into a unit containing a reed or membrane. From here a tube is passed into the mouth, where the sound

produced when lung air passes over the reed or membrane can be articulated into speech. The fundamental frequency can be changed by adjusting the tension of the reed, and the volume by changing pressure of expired air. Two types are the Tokyo Pneumatic Artificial Larynx and the Osaka Artificial Larynx. They are rarely used in the United Kingdom but further details regarding their construction and use can be found in **Salmon and Goldstein** (1978).

2   *The intra-oral electronic larynx* is made up of a battery-powered unit producing a tone which is then transmitted along a plastic tube which is inserted into the mouth (usually into the corner) and between the teeth so that the sound is directed up into the oral cavity and then articulated for speech. Designs vary; the on/off control may be near the mouth-piece, as with the Cooper-Rand Electronic Speech Aid, or on the generator itself, as in the oral adaptation of the Jedcom Electronic Larynx. Adaptations can be made for 'no hands' use of some models (eg. Cooper-Rand) for use by laryngectomees who need both hands free at work or who are unable to use the standard switches. Volume and fundamental frequency can be adjusted. Power is supplied by recharge-able or standard batteries. Some models have slightly rigid mouth tubes which retain an appropriate angle, as opposed to the more flexible tubes.

   The most commonly used devices in the United Kingdom are the Cooper-Rand Electronic Speech Aid and oral adaptations of the Servox Electronic Speech Aid and the Jedcom Electronic Larynx.

3   *The neck-type electronic larynx* consists of a diaphragm of rubber, plastic or metal which is set into vibration by a battery-powered motor usually enclosed in a cylindrical case below the diaphragm. Batteries may be standard or rechargeable, and some models (eg. Servox Intone) may be recharged by replacing the complete unit in a charger without removing the battery. Designs vary, but the sound produced is transmitted into the vocal tract by holding the head of the aid against the neck or cheek skin, so that the sound waves pass through the tissues into the tract to be articulated into speech. On/off switches are usually on the body of the aid and most models can produce a variety of fundamental frequencies and volume of sound. Weight and size vary from model to model, as do construction, sophistication, robustness, cost and reliability!

   The most commonly used models in the United Kingdom include the Servox Artificial Larynx, Jedcom Electronic Speech Aid, Jedcom Artificial Larynx (previously the Bart's model) and the Rexton Laryn-gophone. (*See Useful Addresses for suppliers.*)

Therapy Using Artificial Larynges

The following information relates only to the electronic artificial larynges.

   Salmon (1986c) outlined eight areas which should be worked on when introducing the laryngectomee to a speech aid:

1   Selection
2   Demonstration and acceptability
3   Placement
4   On/off timing
5   Articulation
6   Phrasing
7   Inflection
8   Loudness

They should be considered carefully as they play an important part in the ultimate success or failure of the therapeutic intervention. Let us look at these areas in more detail:

1 Selection

The clinician should ideally have a selection of aids available for the laryngectomee to try out. Many laryngectomees (and clinicians) are biased by experience – that is, only considering models which have been successful in the past.

Financial constraints may prevent the clinician from holding a supply of demonstration aids within the department, but it may be possible to arrange for the laryngectomee to try out another laryngectomee's aid or, in the United Kingdom, to visit a Communication Aids Centre (*see Useful Addresses*) where a range of different aids will be available. When using another laryngectomee's aid, it is essential that the clinician maintains an appropriate degree of hygiene – especially with intra-oral aids – and mouth-pieces should be changed for each individual.

Size and weight should be assessed and the laryngectomee advised to use the aid in the non-dominant hand so that the dominant hand is free. Where a laryngectomee is frail, the heavier models may be unsuitable. Likewise, a robust model would be required for a laryngectomee hoping to return to work.

Power source: some laryngectomees cannot cope with recharging batteries, although models where the complete aid is placed in the charger may alleviate this problem.

Neck or intra-oral type? The intra-oral type can usually be used in intensive care once the laryngectomee is conscious and keen to communicate. Ex-pipe smokers adapt to this type of aid very quickly, and have little difficulty in adjusting articulation to compensate for the mouth-piece being between the teeth. Heavy doses of radiation may result in neck tissue which is scarred, thickened or anaesthetised, leading to subsequent problems in placement of the neck-type aid. However placement may be more successful on the cheek (see below). Excess production of saliva post-operatively may result in the intra-oral aid becoming affected by saliva moving down the mouth-piece – despite the saliva guard – and changing to a neck-type aid may be advisable.

2 Demonstration and Acceptability

Before the demonstration, the clinician must be fully conversant with the aid and its functions. The batteries should be fully charged, and the volume and frequency levels set at an appropriate level for one-to-one conversation.

Salmon (1986c) emphasised the need for the clinician to treat the aid with respect, by using the appropriate terms – artificial larynx, or electronic speech aid, not 'buzzer', 'noise-maker' or some other negative term. The acceptability of the sound produced for the laryngectomee and family can be affected by the clinician's attitude.

When demonstrating the aid for the first time, it may help to 'test' the aid against the hand, to accustom the listeners to the sound that is to be produced, before using it on the neck, or in the mouth.

The clinician should explain the principle behind the aid's use, and explain that it is merely a substitute for the missing 'sound source' for speech, and will not be a complete communication replacement. (One of the author's patients was heard describing his aid to another laryngectomee, expressing wonder at 'how it knows what I want to say'!)

A laryngectomee who is a proficient user of the aid may be able to visit and demonstrate the aid – and, as with oesophageal voice, it is essential that the 'demonstrator' is an efficient speaker, using the aid competently and unobtrusively.

3   Placement

Correct placement of the aid on the neck or in the mouth is essential for success. For the neck-type aid, the aim is to find a soft, pliable area of skin, large enough to place the head of the aid comfortably. The clinician should initially feel the laryngectomee's neck gently, and test any suitable spot by placing the head of the aid firmly against it and switching on. When searching for the correct placement for the aid, the laryngectomee should be encouraged to merely have their mouth open, as if producing an open /a/ sound, but to make no attempt at actually making the sound. Stoma blast should be discouraged from first speech attempts, as this can detract from the general intelligibility of speech.

The correct placement will be obvious immediately, as the /a/ sound will be heard clearly, as if the laryngectomee was producing the sound. Incorrect placement will result in a sound lacking in resonance, or a dull sound which is difficult to locate, or 'leakage' of sound around the head of the aid, resulting in a secondary 'buzz'.

Any spot where pressure triggers coughing or discomfort should not be used.

It is useful then to progress to asking the patient to open and close the lips – /mamamamamam/. These sounds should be heard clearly as well.

The laryngectomee can then be encouraged to try counting up to ten, but articulating the sounds clearly, especially voiceless phonemes (demonstration by the clinician may help here), whilst the clinician ensures continued correct placement of the aid.

Once a successful placement has been established, the laryngectomee can be encouraged to find the same site himself. Where there is a degree of anaesthesia, it may be helpful to mark the spot temporarily. Patients should be encouraged to use the non-dominant hand wherever possible, and to begin monitoring whether there is sound leakage.

Placement of an intra-oral aid should be as comfortable as possible in the mouth, so that there is minimal obstruction of the articulators and therefore of clarity of speech. The tube should be inserted for about 1 to 2 inches into the mouth, and the end of the tube can be cut at an angle of 45° with the open end turned up towards the palate. (This can help prevent tongue or cheek tissue blocking the end of the tube and stopping sound transmission.) A gap between upper side teeth is often a useful place for the tube to be placed so that sound can pass into the oral cavity with minimal obstruction of the teeth.

4   On/off Timing

'Thumb-articulation' training is often required. Most electronic aids require the user to operate the on/off switch using a finger or thumb. In most cases the thumb is more appropriate as the aid can be 'cradled' in the rest of the hand, ensuring its safe and unobtrusive handling.

Some difficulty may be encountered during initial attempts at using the aid, and first speech attempts should be for non-threatening utterances – serial speech, counting etc. Where the aid is switched on too early, a sound will be heard before speech commences and, although later this can be used by proficient speakers to mimic the pausing sound /ɜ/, it should be discouraged initially. Similarly, a delay in switching on results in initial voiced sounds being difficult to comprehend or being perceived as voiceless. Early reminders to 'switch on' only when speech movements are initiated should ensure improved timing, as should encouragement to slow down the rate of speech initially, so that there is time to remember to 'switch on'.

5 Articulation

Where the laryngectomee is being introduced to the artificial larynx at an early stage of rehabilitation, it will be necessary to work on making articulation intelligible now that phonation is no longer via the larynx, and there is no lung air to help produce plosives and stops. Vowels and consonant–vowel combinations should be practised, avoiding voiceless plosives and fricatives:

am	an	all	oil	or	on
ale	aim	aid	eye	isle	I'm
owe	ore	we	wear	wore	um
lie	low	lay	law	lee	loo
me	may	more	my	mere	moor
knee	know	no	nor	name	nail
lame	lane	lone	load	you	

Work on distinguishing between voiced and voiceless sounds should then be carried out without the aid, with the laryngectomee being encouraged to produce clear voiceless plosives and fricatives using only intra-oral changes in pressure and not substituting noisy breathing from the tracheostoma (stoma blast).

Contrasting pairs of words with voiced/voiceless sounds and the same vowel can be practised, with the clinician providing feedback as to whether the sounds are distinct from one another or not:

pie/buy	to/do	cup/cub
cut/gut	bat/bad	tuck/duck
chain/Jane	chess/Jess	chill/Jill
chin/gin	fan/van	vine/fine
vault/fault	file/vile	view/few

With a neck-type aid, it may be possible for the laryngectomee to delay switching on the aid briefly to accentuate voiceless sounds at the beginning of words or before the end of a word ending with a voiceless phoneme, although this is a skill of the refined speaker, not the beginner!

With an intra-oral aid, the laryngectomee will need to compensate for the mouth-tube being in the oral cavity. Initially, articulation may be affected, but with practice the sound distortion can be minimal.

6 Phrasing

Normal inter-word pauses need to be encouraged, so that the laryngectomee does not sound too mechanical. As there is no restriction of speech duration, as with lung-powered speech, it is possible for the artificial larynx speaker to keep talking without pause, and therefore the rules of conversation may need to be explained. The use of interruptors and non-verbal interjections such as /aha/ and voiced agreements should be practised.

With practice, a more natural speaking rhythm can be promoted, so that the tendency to speak in a 'telegraphic' manner is discouraged.

Stress can be added to speech by practising making a short silent pause before a stressed word, and prolonging the voicing on a stressed word fractionally longer.

The rate of speech, as mentioned earlier, should be slightly slower, so that clarity of articulation can be ensured, and so that the listener can become accustomed to the sound being produced.

7 Inflection

Although most electronic speech aids have some adjustments for inflection, few are easily manipulated during connected speech, although recent developments (eg. Servox Intone) have built in intonational changes. The laryngectomee can experiment with producing inflectional changes by moving the neck muscles and 'thinking high' or 'thinking low' and therefore changing the internal contours of the resonators, which will have a corresponding effect on voice quality (**MacCurtain**, 1981).

Changing the pressure on the neck or changing tongue or oral pressure may also change voice quality. Joke-telling is a useful exercise, where the facial expression involved in humour will enable the laryngectomee to experience automatic voice changes.

8 Loudness

The laryngectomee using an electronic speech aid should be discouraged from using the aid at a volume which is inappropriate to the situation. They should be encouraged to consider how they are being perceived by others and, when in the company of other laryngectomees, they should be aware that an over-loud electronic voice may impede the intelligibility of other speakers. This can be a problem with laryngectomees with hearing difficulties, where lack of monitoring of effective volume of speech and effective aid use may impede efficient use.

Quiet speech should be practised, so that in situations where the laryngectomee is required to speak quietly, they will automatically turn down the volume control before speaking.

Telephone use should be practised, and again a slightly reduced volume should be used, so that the person on the receiving end is not deafened! The laryngectomee should be encouraged to hold the telephone mouth-piece well away from the tracheostoma and preferably on the opposite side to the electronic larynx.

As a point of safety, local emergency services – Police, Fire and Ambulance – as well as the laryngectomee's medical centre staff should be familiarised with the sound of the laryngectomee using an electronic aid, so that the laryngectomee is not 'cut off' during speech attempts. Local laryngectomee associations may be involved in familiarisation training for the emergency services, or the clinician can make contact with the individual departments.

Assessment

As with other forms of alaryngeal communication, the clinician should monitor carefully the progress being made in using the aid. The assessments suggested for use with the oesophageal speaker (*see Chapter 5*) can be modified for use with artificial larynx users, or the 'Alaryngeal Speech Checklist' (**Berry, 1976**), devised for this specific group of patients, can be used.

Availability

In the United Kingdom, artificial larynges are available for the laryngectomee on prescription by an ENT consultant. However at times financial constraints may reduce the number of 'spare' aids available. Charitable organisations can often be approached to fund these devices, which serve as the clinician's demonstration aids.

Problems

Although offering almost instant, intelligible speech for the laryngectomee, the use of an artificial larynx should not be seen as a panacea for all difficulties. Aids may not be available or suitable for all laryngectomees, and each user should be carefully monitored and encouraged to become an efficient aid user.

General frailty and/or severe hearing loss may impede success: the laryngectomee may not be able to hold the aid in place; auditory monitoring of correct placement and refinements of speech may be affected. Intention tremor due to associated neurological problems may also affect successful use of the aid.

Severe scarring of the neck may make neck placement impossible and, whereas cheek placement may be possible, swelling in this area may impede transmission of sound. Extensive oral surgery and excess production of saliva may also impede use of an intra-oral aid and clarity of articulation.

Unfortunately, the mechanical unreliability of certain models causes laryngectomees and clinicians great problems. Laryngectomees should be instructed in the care and everyday maintenance of their aid – contact with water and hard surfaces should be discouraged! In the United Kingdom, they should be instructed to return the aid to the department, should any fault occur, and not attempt home repairs. (Another of the author's accident-prone laryngectomees arranged for a friend to put an extra on/off switch onto his aid as the original was not functioning. Needless to say, this invalidated the manufacturers' warranty, and did not solve the problem!)

If an aid is returned as being non-functioning, the clinician should initially suspect battery problems, as rechargeable batteries will eventually lose their ability to maintain a level of charge. When unaccustomed to ordering aids, the clinician is advised to contact a centre experienced in dealing with the different models available and discuss their merits (and faults).

Conclusion

As a planned aid to rehabilitation, an artificial larynx can provide the laryngectomee with quick, intelligible speech soon after surgery, and can be used as a complementary communication method, along with oesophageal speech. It should not be seen as being used only in cases of failure to acquire oesophageal voice.

CHAPTER 8
SURGICAL VOICE RESTORATION I: EVALUATION & ASSESSMENT

CHAPTER 8
SURGICAL VOICE RESTORATION I: EVALUATION & ASSESSMENT

Introduction

A certain proportion of laryngectomees will, for one reason or another, fail to acquire or use oesophageal voice as a useful method of communication post-operatively.

As indicated in *Chapter 6*, reported percentages of failure to acquire oesophageal voice vary from 43 per cent (**King *et al.***, 1968) to 98 per cent (**Hunt**, 1964) with an average of 64–9 per cent (**Snidecor**, 1975). There have been examples of surgeons attempting to overcome this difficulty surgically almost since the beginnings of laryngectomy as a recognised procedure.

The essential objective of Surgical Voice Restoration (SVR) is the re-creation of the physiological situation where air expired from the lungs generates and controls the voice, even after removal of the larynx.

Historical Background

Today's SVR methods have their origins in experimental procedures attempted by Bilroth and Gussenbauer in 1873. These resulted in a certain amount of intelligible speech but the prosthesis was uncomfortable and saliva leakage was a problem. As a result the fistula was repaired and oesophageal speech became the accepted goal for laryngectomees.

SVR was then limited to a few scattered experiments; for example, in 1935, Guttman created a crude vocal fistula between the trachea and the oesophagus using a diathermy needle – this was a forerunner of today's tracheo-oesophageal puncture techniques of **Singer *et al.***, (1981).

In the 1950s SVR came to the fore again, with the work of Briani in Italy and Conley in the United States. Briani used an external vocal fistula and devised a connecting prosthesis with manual control of phonatory air. Conley attempted to create an internal tracheo-oesophageal fistula, using mucous membrane, skin or vein grafts. There was some temporary success with voicing, but there were problems maintaining a patent fistula – some became blocked and others leaked.

In 1965, Asai reported on a surgical procedure involving the construction of a tracheo-hypopharyngeal fistula, and this was an important landmark – some of his patients are still alive today and, following Asai, SVR became popular, with important improvements in safety, reliability and avoidance of complications, especially leakage of saliva.

At present, in the United Kingdom, the procedure which is most popular is derived from the Blom–Singer procedure. Although other techniques and prostheses are being used, in general terms, a clinician working outside a specialist centre is most likely to be asked to deal with laryngectomees who have had a Blom–Singer prosthesis fitted. Detailed descriptions of other SVR procedures can be found in texts such as **Edwards** (1980).

In the past, laryngectomees were mostly considered for this form of SVR as a secondary procedure carried out some time after the initial laryngectomy. Now, however, some centres are carrying out puncture as a primary procedure – at the same time as the removal of the larynx. Throughout this text, the information given will relate to SVR as a secondary procedure, but it would also apply to a primary procedure, apart from obvious exceptions such as pre-procedure assessment.

The Procedure

Technically the Blom–Singer procedure is categorised as a tracheo-oesophageal puncture technique requiring a valved prosthesis. (This category would also include the Panje voice button, the Bivona series of voice restoration products and other, more recent developments such as the Groningen Button, which, at the time of writing, is fitted during initial surgery.)

Figure 4 *Voice prosthesis in place – respiration*

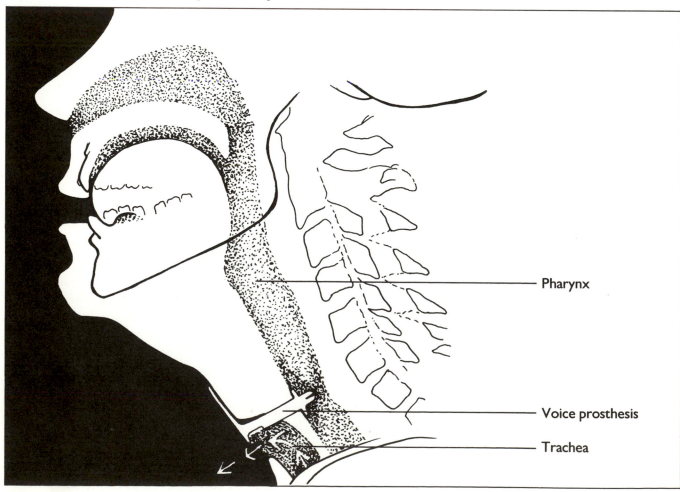

Pharynx

Voice prosthesis

Trachea

The surgical procedure involves constructing an internal fistula between the trachea and the oesophagus. This fistula is kept open by the presence of a small unobtrusive prosthesis with a one-way valve to prevent fluid leakage through the fistula (*see Figure 4*).

Control of phonatory air-flow is by using the finger (or an externally fitted tracheostoma valve) to occlude the tracheostoma, with air being shunted into the oesophagus below the level of the P–E segment. Lung-powered oesophageal voice is then produced (*see Figure 5*).

The surgery involved is relatively simple, with a fistula being created between the trachea and the oesophagus under general anaesthetic, and kept open by the insertion of a catheter which is left in place for 36–48 hours. After this time the catheter can be removed and the prosthesis inserted.

Figure 5 **Voice prosthesis in place – phonation**

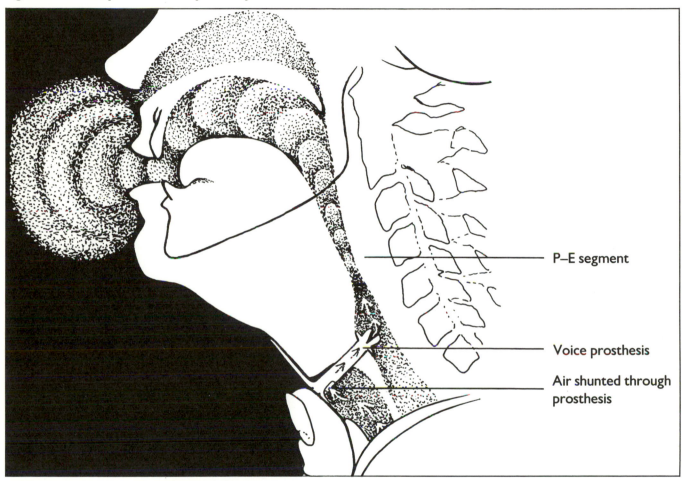

P–E segment

Voice prosthesis

Air shunted through prosthesis

The Clinician's Role

The clinician's role in SVR is an important one, involving all stages from patient selection through to post-procedure therapy. It would be an unwise decision for a surgeon to carry out these procedures without consultation with the clinician, who is, likewise, unable to carry out the procedures without the co-operation of medical colleagues.

Patient Selection

This is probably one of the most important aspects of SVR, involving the complete rehabilitation team – surgeon, clinician, radiologist, nursing and junior medical staff. Careful selection is probably the single most important factor influencing the success or otherwise of the procedure. No laryngectomee should be taken on for SVR without undergoing careful selection (**Cheesman** *et al.*, 1985; **Perry and Edels,** 1985; **Perry** *et al.*, 1987).

The assessment of suitability of a laryngectomee to undergo SVR should involve the surgeon, radiologist and clinician, and should include a videofluoroscopic examination of the structure and function of the vocal tract. (This is described in *Chapter 6*.) The role of the tonic P–E segment in successful SVR is emphasised by **Perry** (1988b).

The results of the videofluoroscopy examination and other important selection criteria can be included on an evaluation sheet such as the one shown in *Figure 6*. The following headings refer to questions on the evaluation.

Figure 6   **Surgical Voice Restoration – assessment**

Name _____ **Unit no** _____
Date of evaluation _____

Results of Insufflation Test _____
_____
_____

General Considerations
  1   Is patient unhappy with present mode of communication? _____
  2   Is patient intelligible to the average listener? _____
  3   Is speech acceptable for patient's needs? _____
  4   Has patient recovered from initial surgery? _____
  5   Is patient disease-free at present? _____
  6   Is patient physically stable? _____
  7   Is patient capable of caring for stoma and prosthesis? _____
  8   Is patient motivated to undergo SVR? _____
  9   Is size of tracheostoma adequate? _____
 10   Is tracheostoma free from ulceration? _____
 11   Check for chronic tracheitis _____
 12   Check tracheostoma position – not behind manubrium _____
 13   Check trachea is not arched above level of stoma _____
 14   Is visual dexterity adequate? _____
 15   Is manual dexterity adequate for self-care? _____
 16   Check for severe arthritis _____
 17   Is patient generally reliable (eg. attending appointments and carrying out
       instructions)? _____
 18   Check for unplanned fistulae or strictures _____
 19   Check sensitivity of stoma _____
 20   Check for occupational constraints for prosthesis use _____
       _____
 21   Is family aware of implications of procedure? _____
 22   Is patient able to attend follow-up clinics? _____

Evaluation carried out by _____ (ENT)
                          _____ (Sp Th)

Recommendations _____
_____
_____
_____

© Eryl Evans, 1990

Results of Insufflation Test

An important aspect of selection for SVR is the result of the insufflation or Taub test (**Taub and Bugner**, 1973), which involves a catheter being inserted into the oesophagus via the nasal cavity to a level below the P–E segment. (This is usually at about the level of the tracheostoma externally.) When carried out during videofluoroscopy, the passage of the catheter via the pharynx can be seen, and the level of the tracheostoma is marked externally, using a radio-opaque marker on the skin.

Air is then blown gently into the oesophagus via the catheter, and this should result in oesophageal voice being produced as the air moves back up and out past the P–E segment. A recent development uses a tracheostoma valve fitted externally which enables the laryngectomee to self-insufflate.

It may be necessary to move the catheter up and down slightly in order to find optimum voicing, and when voice is produced easily the laryngectomee can be encouraged to count gently but without attempting to produce oesophageal voice themselves, merely 'shaping' the sound produced by the insufflation. Possible results of the insufflation include the following:

(a) *Oesophageal voice is produced easily and the quality is acceptable.* When this occurs, it can be seen during the videofluoroscopy that there is a P–E segment capable of producing oesophageal voice. (There have been instances of laryngectomees producing a 'false positive' result, but in general, a positive test suggests a P–E segment functioning well for sound.)

(b) *Oesophageal voice is produced easily, but quality is poor, producing a 'whispery' or 'gurgly' sound.* This suggests that there is too little resistance in the P–E segment (also known as a hypotonic segment). This is not always a contraindication for SVR, as digital pressure on the outside of the neck may result in increased resistance and improved oesophageal voice. Following SVR, increased external pressure can be achieved by wearing a pressure band around the neck, either custom-made, using a band of webbing or elasticated material, fastened using Velcro at the back, or a commercially produced one, such as the Dan Kelly Pressure Band.

A poor-quality voice during insufflation may also be produced if the catheter is above the P–E segment, ie in the hypopharynx, and the sound produced is therefore not true oesophageal voice. This may occur as a result of inexperience of how far the catheter needs to be inserted, or where the laryngectomee has a particularly long neck; inserting the catheter deeper may result in improved voicing. Carrying out the insufflation under videofluoroscopy enables the position of the catheter tip to be seen.

(c) *Oesophageal voice is produced briefly, then ceases.* Where oesophageal voice is produced and then stops, even though air is still being introduced into the oesophagus, this may be because there is too much resistance in the P–E segment (ie a hypertonic segment). During phonation testing, only one or two words are produced (**Perry and Edels,** 1985). Singer and Blom suggest that, when this is apparent, the surgeon injects a nerve-blocking agent, such as Novocaine, into the inferior constrictor muscle, and five minutes later the insufflation test is repeated. With the spasm temporarily removed, voicing is usually successful, and they suggest that selective myotomy of the constrictor muscles is carried out in addition to tracheo-oesophageal puncture (**Singer and Blom**, 1981). Where the hypertonicity is not severe, the laryngectomee may be able to produce satisfactory voice by using a low-pressure prosthesis, which opens at a much lower air pressure, and may not trigger the hyptertonicity.

(d) *No oesophageal voice is produced.* This could be due to a number of factors, the most common being spasm of the P–E segment which results in total resistance to the flow of air. The laryngectomee may sense air moving down into the stomach and feel discomfort in the oesophagus. During videofluoroscopic examination the spasm may be visible, as there may be pooling of the contrast material above the segment, and the passage of air out of the oesophagus can be seen to be restricted. The laryngectomee may complain of swallowing problems, and the passage of the bolus of contrast material during the barium swallow may be slow, or be seen as a 'squirting' movement as it passes the segment.

A permanent oesophageal stricture may be present, especially if inserting the catheter into the oesophagus proves difficult. A stricture should be visible during routine examination of the pharynx as well as during videofluoroscopy and is seen as a permanent fibrous barrier during swallowing and speech attempts, as opposed to a hypertonic P–E segment which is usually only apparent during attempts at voicing. An oesophageal stricture must be removed surgically before successful oesophageal voice can be produced.

Other, less common deterrents to a positive Taub test may be trauma to the P–E segment or reaction to the insertion of the catheter – this should not occur where the catheter is inserted gently, by an experienced person. It is also wise to check that the catheter is not defective – a blocked catheter would result in no air being introduced into the oesophagus! When air is being introduced, it is essential that the laryngectomee does not attempt to produce oesophageal voice independently, as this may interfere with the results of the insufflation.

General Considerations

A positive Taub test is one selection criterion for SVR; other considerations include the following:

Is the patient unhappy with the present mode of communication?
Is the patient motivated to undergo SVR?

The ultimate decision as to whether to carry out SVR should lie with the laryngectomee, and where they are quite satisfied with their communication, even though it may not be 'perfect', their wishes must be respected. The clinician and surgeon may wish to suggest SVR, and explain the procedure and its implications, but the choice must lie with the laryngectomee.

Is the patient intelligible to the average listener?
Is speech acceptable for the patient's needs?

Although the standard of oesophageal speech (or other form of communication) achieved by the laryngectomee may not be superior, it may be more than adequate for their particular needs and circumstances. Where the laryngectomee is intelligible to family, carers and friends, and they are happy with their mode of communication, then again the choice of SVR must be theirs.

Has the patient recovered from initial surgery?
Check for unplanned fistulae or strictures

In the United Kingdom, the majority of cases are still considered for SVR as a secondary procedure, that is some time after the laryngectomy. However, the reader is referred to studies of SVR as a primary procedure. Where it is a secondary procedure, the patient must have recovered physically and psychologically from the initial surgery. They must have had time to become accustomed to being a laryngectomee, and must be physically capable of undergoing the puncture technique. Where there are healing or other post-operative problems, fistulae or strictures, resulting in swallowing and feeding difficulties, it is obviously unwise to submit the oesophagus and surrounding area to additional pressures.

Is the patient disease-free at present?
Check for chronic tracheitis.

Generally speaking, the laryngectomee should be free from disease. Where it is known that malignancy has recurred, it is usually wise to work on achieving effective communication by some other method than SVR. Chronic chest disease or tracheitis can also be contraindications for SVR, as the increase in mucus production can affect successful maintenance of the prosthesis.

Is the patient physically stable?

The immediate post-operative period is obviously one of great change for the laryngectomee, where the body is recovering from surgical trauma and the altered functions for breathing and communication. The patient must be stable following surgery or post-operative radiotherapy before being considered for SVR.

Is the patient capable of caring for stoma and prosthesis?
Is visual dexterity adequate?
Is manual dexterity adequate for self-care?
Check for severe arthritis.

The initial fitting of the voice prosthesis and instruction in caring for it are the responsibility of the clinician, but in most cases it is the laryngectomee who must be responsible for continuing this on discharge home. There must be sufficient visual and manual dexterity for the laryngectomee to be able to clean and change the prosthesis successfully. Hygiene is imperative in order to maintain a healthy area around the stoma and puncture site. The prosthesis, its inserter and the puncture site are small, and it would be difficult for a person with poor visual and manual dexterity to cope. However it may be possible to instruct a relative or other carer to look after the prosthesis, or for the laryngectomee to attend at the out-patients department where distances permit.

Is the size of tracheostoma adequate?
Is the tracheostoma free from ulceration?
Check tracheostoma position – not behind manubrium.
Check trachea is not arched above the stoma.

The Blom–Singer prosthesis is fitted into a puncture situated in the wall of the trachea, and therefore the retaining strap protrudes through the tracheostoma. A very small stoma would naturally be occluded to some degree by the presence of the prosthesis, and this must not be to such an extent that breathing is affected. Where the stoma is deemed too small to accommodate the prosthesis safely, stoma revision may be necessary to increase its size. It is also more difficult to carry out the puncture when the stoma is behind the manubrium, or the trachea is arched up above the level of the stoma. In such a case, it may be necessary for the prosthesis to be modified (**Perry, Cheesman and Eden**, 1982). An ulcerated tracheostoma must be treated before tracheo-oesophageal puncture is considered, as fitting and changing the prosthesis may exacerbate the ulceration.

Is the patient generally reliable (eg. attending appointments and carrying out instructions)?
Is the patient able to attend follow-up clinics?
Is the patient's family aware of the implications of the procedure?

The laryngectomee cannot undertake SVR and then be expected to be able to use and care for the prosthesis without monitoring by professionals. Where a patient is unable to attend clinics because of travel or time constraints, alternative arrangements must be made for follow-up appointments. It may be possible to refer them on to a centre nearer their home, in which case the clinician in that area needs to be notified of the transfer, and be prepared to take on the laryngectomee and capable of managing the voice prosthesis. In addition, the family or carers need to be aware of the implications of the procedure, how to care for the prosthesis, and what to do in an emergency. Written instructions on care of the prosthesis should be given out and explained thoroughly, in order to prevent unnecessary closure of the puncture should the prosthesis be dislodged. (*See page 73, 'Fitting the Prosthesis'*.)

Check sensitivity of stoma.

Where the tracheostoma is excessively sensitive, this needs to be progressively desensitised before puncturing. This can be done by inserting a stoma button for increasing periods. It may be necessary for the surgeon to anaesthetise the stoma initially, but eventually the laryngectomee should be able to tolerate the stoma button without the violent reactions associated with a sensitive stoma.

Check for occupational constraints for prosthesis use.

On its own, the Blom–Singer prosthesis is used by the laryngectomee occluding the tracheostoma with a finger. Where a laryngectomee needs to have two hands free during work, a tracheostoma valve, which enables the prosthesis to be used 'hands-free', may have to be considered.

Where the evaluation has shown that the laryngectomee would be suitable for SVR, the next stage is for the surgeon to arrange admission for SVR. In theory, this can be carried out as an out-patient procedure, but in the United Kingdom it is usual for the laryngectomee to be admitted, ensuring that the clinician has the opportunity for intensive instruction in the management of the prosthesis. Management and therapy procedures are discussed in the next chapter.

CHAPTER 9
SURGICAL VOICE RESTORATION II: MANAGEMENT & THERAPY

CHAPTER 9
SURGICAL VOICE RESTORATION II: MANAGEMENT & THERAPY

Pre-puncture

When the laryngectomee is awaiting SVR it is advisable to make a permanent recording of their communication, so that this may be compared post-puncture. A video recording of the laryngectomee should be made, including reading and conversation as well as repetition of phrases and serial speech. Where video recording is unavailable, a good quality audio recording should be made, along with an objective assessment of speech abilities, for example 'Oesophageal Voice Assessment' (**Gardner**, 1971) or 'Alaryngeal Speech Checklist' (**Berry**, 1976).

The laryngectomee should also be given further information about the procedure and time-scale of events. The video 'Voice Your Choice' is available on free loan, for up to one month, from the Speech Therapy Department, Charing Cross Hospital, London, for pre-operative viewing by potential SVR patients. This covers all aspects of the procedure, comparing SVR with conventional oesophageal speech and makes an unbiased comparison of both.

Fitting the Prosthesis

Detailed instructions for fitting and changing prostheses are not included in this chapter, as it is recommended that the clinician receives thorough training, preferably at a specialist centre, where theory is supplemented by invaluable practical experience of fitting and changing prostheses.

The clinician is responsible for fitting the correct size of prosthesis (**Bosone**, 1986), and at no time should the fistula be left open for more than a short period of time as closure occurs rapidly – within minutes the fistula will seem tighter; after 30 minutes, reinsertion of the prosthesis will be difficult, while the puncture will almost certainly have closed completely after 24 hours.

It is usually easier for the clinician to occlude the stoma for the initial attempts at voicing, and the laryngectomee should resist the temptation to exhale forcibly, and be instructed to breathe out gently. Voicing should then be attempted for an open vowel, followed by serial counting or going through the days of the week. Patients should be discouraged from forcing the sound out, or using any other method for producing oesophageal voice, such as injection.

Where no oesophageal voice is produced after a number of attempts, the clinician should follow the 'troubleshooting' procedure:

1   *Prosthesis in, no voice.*   Try open tract voicing. Remove the prosthesis briefly, occlude the stoma and attempt voicing. If oesophageal voice is produced, the problem is due to prosthesis problems, or the way in which it is being used. Check:

(a)   that the slit at the end of the prosthesis is open. If it is closed, it may be opened by gently squeezing the tip of the prosthesis or by using a razor blade to gently open the slit. If the prosthesis is severely defective, a new prosthesis should be used.

(b)   the size of the prosthesis. If it is too long, the tip of the prosthesis may be touching the posterior pharyngeal wall; this also occurs if too much pressure is exerted on the stoma during occlusion. There should be sufficient pressure only to prevent air escape. Where the laryngectomee senses the prosthesis touching the pharyngeal wall, a smaller prosthesis should be fitted. The laryngectomee may require a shorter prosthesis with time, as the fistula becomes more established.

Conversely, if the prosthesis is too short, there may be voicing initially, but, after a time, there is a danger that the oesophageal opening of the fistula will close, as the prosthesis is not keeping the channel open for the whole length of the tract. Once the prosthesis is in place, there should be resistance to gentle tugging on the bottom of the retaining strap. Where the prosthesis moves out, it is likely that the prosthesis is too short, and a longer one should be fitted. As the prosthesis is radio-opaque, an X-ray can be taken to check that it is in the correct position.

(c)   that the laryngectomee is breathing out! Often, as soon as the stoma is occluded, they automatically hold their breath, as they believe there is 'no way out' for the air. It may be advisable for the clinician to occlude the stoma for initial voicing attempts, where air pressure should be felt behind the occluding thumb or finger.

(d)   the quality of voice produced. If it is very weak or 'whispery', this may be due to an inadequate P–E segment. This should have been identified during the pre-operative evaluation, and digital pressure on the neck externally should be used to increase the resistance of the segment. Care should be taken that digital pressure is not excessive, blocking the pharyngeal lumen, and preventing voice production. A wet 'gurgly' sound may be produced if there is excessive saliva in the oesophagus, and the laryngectomee should be encouraged to swallow or expectorate this saliva.

2   *Prosthesis in, no voice, prosthesis out, no voice.*   Where there is no voicing on open tract phonation, this is usually owing to spasm of the P–E segment or an oesophageal stricture. These should have been identified during the pre-operative evaluation, and managed accordingly. Where a hypertonic segment is suspected post-puncture, it may be possible to use a low-pressure valve, which requires less expiratory air pressure to function, and this reduced pressure may not stimulate the hypertonicity as much as a

regular duckbill valve. Where this is unsuccessful, a myotomy may need to be considered.

A similar result will occur if a prosthesis which is too short has been inserted, in which case the pharyngeal end of the tract may have healed over. This can be checked by gently inserting the catheter into the puncture site, when it should eventually be felt touching the posterior wall of the pharynx. Where the puncture site has obviously begun to heal, the surgeon needs to be contacted and a re-puncture considered, or dilation may be possible in the clinic, using urethral dilators, without the need for repeat anaesthesia, if the closure is attended to promptly.

Patient Instruction

When the prosthesis has been fitted successfully, the clinician should instruct the laryngectomee in its care and fitting. Written instructions should accompany practical demonstration and experience. Patients should also be given a spare prosthesis and catheter, and advised of the procedure to carry out if having problems with their prosthesis. They should be encouraged to carry some form of written information at all times, so that the prosthesis is not removed unnecessarily during an emergency. An example of written instructions which could be given is shown in *Figure 7*.

Figure 7 **Care of your voice prosthesis**

1 Always make sure that either the voice prosthesis or the red rubber catheter is in the fistula at all times.
2 Always carry your catheter with you. If left open, the fistula will start closing within minutes, and make it very difficult, if not impossible, to reinsert the prosthesis.
3 Always check that the prosthesis is in correctly. If you tug gently at the bottom of the retaining strap the prosthesis should not move out of the fistula more than very slightly.
4 Before changing the prosthesis, check that you have everything you need: catheter, prosthesis, tape, cotton buds etc.
5 It is not necessary to remove the prosthesis daily, just clean it in position. If it seems very dirty, remove it and immediately replace it with the catheter. Try not to swallow when there is nothing in the fistula.
6 Clean the prosthesis with plenty of warm water and dry it carefully. Do not use very hot water or harsh detergents. Check that the inside of the prosthesis is not blocked.
7 Remove the catheter and replace the prosthesis immediately, using the inserter. Don't panic if it is difficult to insert the prosthesis; just replace the catheter, tape it in place and leave it there for a short while. It should then be easier to reinsert the prosthesis. If not, replace the catheter and contact the hospital.
8 Check that the prosthesis is working by trying to produce voice. Check for leakage by having something to drink.
9 A prosthesis needs replacing when it leaks saliva or fluids. You will notice that you cough after drinking, or you may see drops of liquid around the prosthesis. If changing the prosthesis does not help, contact the hospital.
10 A small amount of blood around the fistula is normal after changing the prosthesis. If bleeding continues, contact the hospital.

IF YOU ARE AT ALL CONCERNED ABOUT CHANGING THE PROSTHESIS – CONTACT THE ENT DEPARTMENT

© Eryl Evans, 1990

Further Therapy

Once a prosthesis has been fitted successfully, the clinician and laryngec-tomee need to work together on the most efficient use of the prosthesis. **Perry** (1983) states that 'It is not adequate to provide a laryngectomee with a new method of voice production . . . and then expect him to "go away and practise".'

There are specific areas of voice and speech production which should be worked on. Perry again suggests that these can be categorised under four headings:

I Valving

The patient has to learn how to use the finger for occluding the stoma. There must be complete occlusion for successful voice production. It is usually necessary to experiment until the laryngectomee discovers the easiest, most consistent method for occlusion. The movement of the hand to occlude should be unobtrusive, and the laryngectomee should practise this, so that distract-ing movements are reduced. Working in front of a mirror may help initially, although they should eventually aim to be able to feel when the stoma is occluded. Some prefer to use a thumb to occlude, although most men will find their forefinger adequate for occlusion. Where the stoma is large, it is possible to occlude the stoma using a handkerchief made into a pad and placed over the stoma for the appropriate length of time.

Incomplete occlusion leads to air escape around the stoma, and this reduces the intelligibility of speech; on the other hand, if the laryngectomee occludes the stoma with too much force, the tip of the prosthesis is pushed back against the posterior oesophageal wall and the air cannot pass through. Therefore it is useful to go through a series of valving 'drills' emphasising gentle, but efficient occlusion:

> Breathe in
> Occlude stoma
> Voicing for /a/
> Remove finger
> Breathe in

The laryngectomee should be encouraged to take gentle breaths in, and not to expect to be able to speak continuously on one breath. This co-ordination of breathing with speech attempts may take a little time to become familiar again, especially if there has been some success with oesophageal voice, where speech is mostly dissociated from breathing.

2 Articulation

As with conventional oesophageal speech, articulation needs to be open and slow. Where the laryngectomee has experienced oesophageal speech or working with an electronic larynx, this should be established, but this may need to be reiterated when starting work using the prosthesis, and lists of minimal pairs worked through.

3 Rate

The rate of speech needs to be slightly slower in order to accommodate the time needed to co-ordinate air intake and voicing, and also for clear articulation.

4   Phrasing

As mentioned above, the laryngectomee may try to get too many words out on one intake of air. Although the availability of air is greatly increased owing to the use of lung air, they should be discouraged from trying to use up all the air for each speech attempt. A reminder to remove their finger when breathing in may also be required. Reading passages marked off into phrases of suitable lengths can be practised, as well as reading without attempting to produce oesophageal voice by any previously attempted methods, such as injection.

Tracheostoma Valve

In 1983, a tracheostoma valve was made available which can be used where manual occlusion of the stoma is inconvenient. This valve is inserted into a plastic housing which is fixed around the tracheostoma using special adhesive tape and liquid. A diaphragm in the valve enables air to be taken in and out for respiration, but, during speech attempts, the diaphragm closes and air is shunted through the voice prosthesis. Diaphragms of different thicknesses are available, and the most appropriate sensitivity should be chosen so that breathing for routine physical activity, such as walking upstairs, is not impeded. As with fitting the prosthesis, it is advisable that the clinician is trained in fitting and instructing the laryngectomee in using the tracheostoma valve.

Benefits of SVR

Following insertion of a Blom–Singer or similar voice prosthesis, there are definite advantages for the laryngectomee, in that voice production is quick and, in most cases, there is little difficulty in becoming proficient at using the prosthesis for speech.

Voicing is once again 'lung-powered', and therefore louder and longer utterances can be produced. The procedure is also reversible, should the laryngectomee experience problems, as the removal of the prosthesis without replacing a stenting catheter will result in the fistula closing within 24 hours in most cases.

Intelligible speech is possible within a very short time and, in the case of SVR carried out as a primary procedure (that is at the time of laryngectomy), the patient can be expected to go home with intelligible speech. Results with SVR being carried out as a primary procedure are promising, and **Perry** (1988b) suggests that this may be the result of 'careful planning of pharyngeal closure by the surgeon after removal of the larynx'. It may be that, in the future, more and more prospective laryngectomees will be offered SVR as a primary procedure, at the same time as laryngectomy. However the procedure must rely on careful patient selection and co-operation between all members of the rehabilitation team.

Problems with SVR

SVR is not suitable for all laryngectomees, and even following careful selection some laryngectomees may fail to become proficient speakers. **Perry** (1988a) notes that some patients were dissatisfied with the quality of the voice produced, others in the author's experience have found maintenance of the prosthesis difficult, as the result either of deteriorating faculties (visual acuity, general health) or of problems with fungal infections around the prosthesis. Some patients have removed the prosthesis 'accidentally' and left the puncture site open so that closure has taken place, and not requested re-puncturing. In all cases, the feelings and wishes of the individual should be respected, regardless of the clinician's or other staff's feelings.

Note: Where SVR is unavailable at the laryngectomee's own hospital, it is possible for them to request assessment for the procedure at a specialist centre, in which case the clinician is advised to liaise closely with this centre to ensure successful use and maintenance of the prosthesis on discharge home.

CHAPTER 10
GENERAL INFORMATION & FURTHER MANAGEMENT

CHAPTER 10
GENERAL INFORMATION & FURTHER MANAGEMENT

Introduction

Working with laryngectomees involves the clinician in much more than working on speech rehabilitation in isolation. In the 'Inventory for the Assessment of Laryngectomee Rehabilitation', **La Borwit** (1976) emphasises the fact that the person who is best informed about all aspects of their condition is 'the most likely to achieve successful rehabilitation'.

In order to facilitate maximum rehabilitation, the clinician needs to be aware of the wide range of issues which may affect the success or otherwise of rehabilitation. Some of these will be discussed in this chapter. The reader is also referred to the informative chapter by **Darvill** in Edels (1983), and the texts written by **Seddon** (date not known) and **Keith** *et al*. (1984).

Stoma Care

Post-operatively, often one of the most difficult aspects of laryngectomy for the patient and carer to cope with is the presence of a permanent tracheostoma. The permanent nature of this neck opening is sometimes difficult for the laryngectomee to comprehend and accept, and therefore caring for the stoma needs to be approached in a sensitive and informed way by all staff. The initial information regarding stoma care may be given by the nursing staff or by physiotherapists during the stay in hospital. However the clinician, in regular contact post-operatively and on discharge home, is in an ideal situation to reinforce this information and ensure that an appropriate standard of care is being maintained.

Many different stoma covers are available – both commercially and following laryngectomees' own designs. It is essential for both health and social acceptance that the stoma is kept covered, especially in dry, dusty or extremely cold conditions. Air taken in pre-operatively is filtered, humidified and warmed by passing via the nasal or oral cavities and the whole length of the vocal tract before entering the lungs, whereas, post-operatively, most of the tract is absent, and unfiltered, cold air can be taken in almost directly into the lungs.

In the United Kingdom, there are three main types of commercially available stoma covers:

The Buchanan Laryngectomy Protector – a foam filter within a cotton cellular bib which is attached around the neck with tapes. It can be washed a limited number of times before the foam becomes discoloured. It is available on prescription in the United Kingdom. (*See Useful Addresses for suppliers.*)

Laryngofoam Filter – small squares of foam (approx. 5 cm × 6 cm) with a hypoallergenic adhesive strip along the top edge. These are affixed just above the stoma so that the foam covers the opening. They are disposable, and the laryngectomee needs to carry spares, as they may need to be replaced during the day. Before fixing them to the skin, the laryngectomee should ensure that the surrounds of the stoma are clean and dry, as moisture would affect the adhesive quality of the strip. They are available on prescription in the United Kingdom. (*See Useful Addresses for suppliers.*)

Romet Laryngectomy Collar – a cotton 'turtle-neck'-style cover which is fastened at the back of the neck using Velcro. Collars come in assorted colours and, when worn under an open-neck shirt, give the impression of a turtle-neck sweater. They are washable, but not available on prescription. (*See Useful Addresses for suppliers.*)

Some laryngectomees may prefer to use squares of gauze held in place by tape sewn or folded over the upper edge, or to have one crocheted in cotton. A scarf or cravat may also be worn to conceal the stoma, although it is advisable for the material to be protected from mucus expelled during coughing.

It is important that the laryngectomee has easy, quick access to the stoma, so any clothing arranged over the stoma should be easily removable. The top or second button of a shirt or blouse can be removed, and sewn onto the outside to give the appearance of being closed, but leaving the opening to the stoma easily accessible. (Where the top button is removed, it may be necessary to replace it with a snap-fastener or small pieces of Velcro in order to keep the collar closed.)

Where the laryngectomee feels uncomfortable having the stoma cover in contact with the stoma, a small wire frame can be purchased which holds the cover away from the stoma. (*See Useful Addresses for suppliers.*)

General Stoma Hygiene

The laryngectomee needs to maintain a suitable level of general hygiene when looking after the stoma. They should be encouraged to cover the stoma with a hand when coughing, and also to develop an efficient, unobtrusive method of clearing the stoma of mucus after coughing. They should be encouraged to carry tissues with them at all times, and it is often useful to include a plastic bag to transport used tissues until a suitable disposal method can be found. It is certainly not necessary to instruct all laryngectomees in such basic details, but, at times, each aspect of stoma care must be covered in detail, as it is for most people a completely unfamiliar procedure which can be distressing and uncomfortable if not carried out correctly.

Humidification may be helpful where the laryngectomee is subjected to dry air, such as in centrally-heated buildings. The use of a moistened stoma cover, or going into a steamy atmosphere (eg. bathroom) may help. Humidification in the bedroom at night may alleviate night-time discomfort.

Crusting of dried mucus around the stoma can cause chapping and discomfort, and this should be avoided by keeping the stoma and surrounding area meticulously clean and by the occasional application of a lubricating jelly (eg. Vaseline). In addition there are commercially available humidifying filters that fit into the tracheostoma tube, or a spray for keeping the stoma moist. (*See Useful Addresses for suppliers.*)

Laryngectomees should be warned of the danger of foreign bodies entering the stoma, and therefore encouraged to keep the opening covered. Stoma buttons may be worn to maintain an easy airway opening, and these are usually supplied by the hospital. The laryngectomee should be instructed in the care and cleaning of the button by the nursing staff before discharge home.

Showering and Bathing

Care must be taken while showering and bathing that water does not enter the tracheostoma (and therefore the trachea), which causes a severe coughing reaction. Some laryngectomees cope by cupping one hand over the stoma, or wearing a damp stoma cover (not the self-adhesive type). There are commercially available shower shields. (*See Useful Addresses for suppliers.*) These are *not* suitable for swimming.

Eating, Taste and Smell

Some laryngectomees experience problems with eating. Some find that food has to be chewed more thoroughly, or that they are restricted to a soft diet. This may be a particular problem where there has been extensive surgery, or damage to, for example, the nerve supply of the tongue. In general, once healing is complete and the oesophagus has adjusted to its new dual role, there should be few problems. Any subsequent difficulties in swallowing should be referred to the medical staff for investigation.

Nutrition may have been affected by the health of the patient pre-operatively, and it is usual for the hospital dietitian to be involved in monitoring post-operative return to adequate nutrition.

A proportion of laryngectomees report an altered sense of taste and smell post-operatively, with the sense of smell being particularly affected as air no longer passes over the sensory cells of the nose during routine inspiration. The sense of smell is also associated with the finer points of taste, and the loss of one sense can affect the other. **Seddon** (date not known) suggests that the sense of smell can be encouraged to be more effective by trying to consciously draw air into the nose 'using something with a strong smell, like an onion, soap etc'.

Bosone (1979) suggests the use of a simple 'nipple tube' for more effective smelling after laryngectomy, where a flexible rubber tube is fitted onto a baby bottle teat (nipple), with one end of the tube being placed in the mouth and held in place between the teeth, and the rubber teat being placed over the tracheostoma. Air can then be redirected via the nose, both for breathing in and breathing out. This improves smelling and can aid with nose-blowing, another function impaired post-laryngectomy. The reader is referred to the original text for detailed instructions for construction and training in its use.

First Aid

Following laryngectomy, any First Aid treatment requiring artificial respiration or resuscitation should be modified to ensure mouth to neck, not mouth to mouth, resuscitation is carried out.

The laryngectomee should be encouraged to carry some form of emergency information at all times, either in the form of emergency pocket cards or an emergency car sticker (available from the National Association of Laryngectomee Clubs (NALC) in the United Kingdom, or the International Association of Laryngectomees (IAL) in the United States), or an emergency bracelet or necklace (eg. Medic Alert).

Hobbies

The laryngectomee should be encouraged, wherever feasible, to maintain an interest in as many of their interests and hobbies as possible. With the obvious exceptions of some water-based sports, most hobbies can and are pursued with great enjoyment by laryngectomees.

Swimming as a hobby was always deemed to be the one form of exercise unavailable to the laryngectomee post-operatively, but, in recent years, the development of swimming aids has made swimming possible. However it must be emphasised that these must only be used under supervision and following training by an approved centre with strict guidelines for use. The laryngectomee who is interested in swimming is advised to contact their national laryngectomee association, such as NALC or IAL.

Air Travel

Air travel should not be a problem for the laryngectomee, once medical clearance for travel has been given. It is advisable to contact the airline before travelling, although most are accustomed to the needs of the laryngec- tomee. The provision of a child's oxygen mask is preferable, as the smaller, softer cuff makes contact with the tracheostoma easier. During flight, humidification is advisable, as dehydration on long flights can result in discomfort.

Social Activities

The laryngectomee should be encouraged to resume their social lives as much as possible, and to avoid withdrawing from social contact. Initial social contacts may be difficult where spoken communication is less than effective, but, in time, and with understanding from friends and associates, the laryngectomee should be able to readjust.

Often the volume of oesophageal voice is inadequate for noisy social gatherings, and where this is a persistent problem for the laryngectomee, added to similar problems at work, they should be offered the provision of an amplifier. There are many different models on the market, and the clinician is advised to experiment with different models so that the one chosen is the most appropriate for the individual. (In the United Kingdom, amplifiers can be prescribed by a consultant surgeon. A range of amplifiers is usually available for trial at Communication Aids Centres.)

Telephone Use

When using the telephone, it is essential for the laryngectomee to take certain precautions to ensure maximum effectiveness. If using oesophageal voice, they should be encouraged to keep the mouth-piece well away from the stoma, at the level of the corner of the mouth, so that sound is directly transmitted into the receiver, and not masked by expired lung air — especially where stoma blast is a problem. Where volume is still inadequate for telephone use, an amplifying telephone can be made available.

Some laryngectomees prefer an artificial larynx for telephone use, and in this case it is again advisable to keep the telephone mouth-piece well away from the stoma. Local emergency services should be advised of the sound of the laryngectomee communicating using an artificial larynx, so that a call is immediately recognised. This may not be a problem in urban areas, but may be in rural situations, where a laryngectomee may provide the first and only experience telephone operators have of understanding alaryngeal speech.

Other laryngectomees prefer to keep a tape recorder near the telephone with a short emergency message on it, which can be played over the telephone when necessary; others again have devised a system of calling for help using specified numbers of telephone rings to a relative or neighbour. (There are commercially available telephone communication devices, and the clinician is advised to contact their local Communication Aids Centre for further details.)

Laryngectomee Clubs

In many areas, groups of laryngectomees have formed themselves into support groups. They meet at regular intervals to enjoy social, informal and formal meetings. In the United Kingdom, most clubs are affiliated to NALC, and they can be contacted for details of club locations. There are national associations in many countries, and details of these can be obtained by contacting the NALC or the IAL in the United States.

Family and Carer Support

Following laryngectomy, it is not the laryngectomee alone who goes through a period of great adjustment, but also the whole network of carers and relatives. Following a time of great emotional and physical tension, it is hardly surprising that strains are put on relationships.

Many spouses report difficulties, with the laryngectomee being self-centred and demanding on discharge home. The change from receiving intensive attention while an in-patient to having to cope at home can be frightening and disorientating for the laryngectomee, but they should be made aware that their spouse has also undergone great emotional stresses and should not be expected to take the place of a whole team of professional carers.

It is often useful for the clinician to contact the spouse independently, to find out how they are coping at home. Many will express great relief at being told that they are not the only ones to experience these problems. Many experience great guilt if they feel irritated by the laryngectomee, as they feel they ought to be 'grateful that they are still alive' but are also finding it very difficult to cope with their spouse, who may be behaving in a completely unfamiliar way. Contact with other spouses before and after the operation may help alleviate this situation, and many spouses are involved in the activities of laryngectomee clubs.

It may be difficult for the laryngectomee or spouse to discuss sexual relationships with any member of the rehabilitation team. During the hospital stay there are so many things to be assimilated, and on discharge home their main contact may be a clinician who is usually female, and often young. It is therefore helpful for the clinician to mention sexual relationships in passing when discussing how most aspects of daily life can be maintained post-laryngectomy. Specific suggestions for coping with problems, such as odour from the stoma and excessive breathing noises, are made in **Keith et al.**, 'Looking Forward . . . A Guidebook for the Laryngectomee' (*see 'Publications' in Useful Addresses*).

The change in family relationships may also be affected if the laryngectomee is no longer the principal wage-earner, and this can often cause problems within the family. Employment and financial difficulties exacerbate tensions and, when these are apparent, the referral to support services (eg. social worker, disablement resettlement officer) should be encouraged.

Terminal Care

It is unfortunate that a proportion of patients will not be cured of cancer following surgery. At some point following treatment the carcinoma may recur to such an extent that further treatment is impossible or inadvisable. It may seem difficult to accept responsibility for those patients in our care for whom we can offer no permanent improvement, but a clinician can offer a great deal to even the terminally ill patient.

Being a regular, friendly visitor can do much to alleviate the loneliness of a patient – even one on a busy hospital ward – and being a familiar face means so much amid strange surroundings. Where the laryngectomee has lost their ability to produce oesophageal voice through disease recurrence, they should be supplied with an artificial larynx or other communication aid. Neck-type artificial larynges may not be suitable where there is swelling and discomfort in the neck, and an intra-oral aid may not be suitable where there has been additional tongue involvement. In these cases a general communication aid, such as a chart or communicator, can be supplied, so that the laryngectomee maintains dignity for as long as possible.

Contact with the family may be difficult when the laryngectomee is dying, but the clinician should not deprive the relatives of the opportunity to share their grief and worries with a familiar face. There are many established grief and bereavement counselling organisations and groups, and the relatives should be encouraged to seek their expert advice where necessary.

The clinician should not be expected to cope alone with all the difficulties encountered by the laryngectomee and their family, but it is essential to be aware of the problems which may occur, so that, as part of the rehabilitation team, they are able to cope and offer the best possible support for all concerned.

APPENDIX
USEFUL ADDRESSES

General Information

Cancer Relief Macmillan Fund,
Anchor House,
15-19 Britten Street,
London SW3 3TZ.

Royal College of Speech and Language Therapists,
7 Bath Place,
Rivington Street,
London EC2A 3DR.

International Association of Laryngectomees (IAL),
American Cancer Society,
777 Third Avenue,
New York NY10017,
USA.

National Association of Laryngectomee Clubs (NALC),
Ground Floor,
6 Rickett Street,
London SW6 1RU.

Communication Aids

Dan Kelly Pressure Band
Dan Kelly,
Speech and Hearing Institute,
1343 Moursund,
Houston,
Texas,
USA.

Servox Artificial Larynx, Amplicord,
Medela Amplifiers, Artificial Larynges, Amplifiers
Kapitex Healthcare Limited,
Kapitex House,
1 Sandbeck Way,
Wetherby,
West Yorkshire LS22 7GH

Medici Amplifier
Ingrams Hearing Aids,
London Road,
Riverhead,
Sevenoaks,
Kent.

Communication Aids Centres (UK)

Charing Cross Hospital (Adults),
Fulham Palace Road,
London W6 8RF.

Frenchay Hospital,
Frenchay,
Bristol BS16 1LE.

Musgrave Park Hospital,
Stockman's Lane,
Belfast B19 7JB.

Rookwood Hospital,
Llandaff,
Cardiff CF5 2YN.

Royal Victoria Infirmary,
Queen Victoria Road,
Newcastle-upon-Tyne NE1 4LP.

Sandwell Centre,
Boulton Road,
West Bromwich B70 6NN.

The Wolfson Centre (Children),
Mecklenburgh Square,
London WC1N 2AP.

General Stoma Care

Wire Cages
Downs Surgical Limited,
Chiron House,
32 New Cavendish Street,
London W1M 8BU.

Rogers Crystal Spray
Frank A Rogers,
1 Beaumont Street,
London W1N 2BU.

Humidifying filter
Portex Limited,
Boundary Road,
Hythe,
Kent CT21 6JL.

Stoma covers
(available on prescription in the community)
Kapitex Healthcare Limited,
Kapitex House,
1 Sandbeck Way,
Wetherby,
West Yorkshire LS22 7GH

Emergency Information Cards/Bracelets

International Association of Laryngectomees (IAL),
American Cancer Society,
777 Third Avenue,
New York NY10017,
USA.

Medic Alert Foundation,
11-13 Clifton Terrace,
London N4.

Medic Alert Foundation,
PO Box 1009,
Turlock,
California 95380,
USA.

National Association of Layngectomee Clubs (NALC),
Ground Floor,
6 Rickett Street,
London SW6 1RU.

Publications and Textbooks

After your Laryngectomy, a Guide for Patient and Family
Valerie Seddon,
Lister Hospital,
Coreys Mill Lane,
Stevenage,
Herts SG1 4AB.

A Handbook for the Laryngectomee,
Robert L Keith,
The Interstate Printers and Publishers Incorporated,
Danville,
Illinois,
USA.

The Artificial Larynx Handbook
S J Salmon, L P Goldstein,
Grune & Stratton Incorporated,
111 Fifth Avenue,
New York NY10003,
USA.

Laryngectomee Rehabilitation
R L Keith, F L Darley,
College-Hill Press Inc.,
PO Box 35728,
Houston,
Texas,
USA.

Laryngectomy and After Laryngectomy
Department of Nursing,
The Royal National Throat, Nose and Ear Hospital,
330 Gray's Inn Road,
London WClX 8DA.

Laryngectomy and what it means to you
Royal College of Speech and Language Therapists,
7 Bath Place,
Rivington Street,
London EC2A 3DR

Laryngectomy: Diagnosis to Rehabilitation
Yvonne Edels (editor),
Croom Helm Limited,
Provident House,
Burrell Row,
Beckenham,
Kent BR3 lAT.

Laryngectomy - your questions answered
Royal Marsden Hospital Patient Information Series,
Haigh and Hochland Limited,
International University Booksellers,
The Precinct Centre,
Oxford Road,
Manchester M13 9QA.

Living with Laryngectomy - audio and slide programme,
Camera Talks Limited,
197 Botley Road,
Oxford OX2 OHE.

Looking Forward... A Guidebook for the Laryngectomee
R L Keith, H C Shane, H L C Coates, K D Devine,
Thieme–Stratton Inc.,
New York,
USA

Self-Help for the Laryngectomee
Edmund Lauder,
115 Whisper Hollow,
San Antonio,
Texas 78238,
USA.

BIBLIOGRAPHY

Bagshaw MJ, 'Rehabilitation of Post-Laryngectomy Patients', *British Journal of Disorders of Communication*, 2, 1967.

Berlin CI, 'Clinical Measurements of Esophageal Speech; I Methodology and Curves of Skill Acquisition', *Journal of Speech and Hearing Disorders*, 28, 1963.

Berry RJ, 'Radiotherapy and Chemotherapy', Edels Y (ed), *Laryngectomy: Diagnosis to Rehabilitation*, Croom Helm, London, 1983.

Berry W, 'Towards Perceptual Reliability and Acceptability', *Proceedings of The Use of the Artificial Larynx in Laryngectomee Rehabilitation*, Rehabilitation Conference, Birmingham, Alabama, 1976.

Bosone ZT, 'A simple device for smelling and nose blowing after Laryngectomy', Lauder E (ed), *Self-Help for the Laryngectomee*, Texas, 1979.

Bosone ZT, 'Troubleshooting after tracheoesophageal fistulization for voice restoration', Shanks JC (ed), *Current Strategies of Rehabilitation of the Laryngectomized Patient*, 7, 1, *Seminars in Speech and Language*, Thieme Inc., New York, 1986.

Cheesman AD, 'Surgical Management of the Patient', Edels Y (ed), *Laryngectomy: Diagnosis to Rehabilitation*, Croom Helm, London, 1983.

Cheesman AD, Knight J, McIvor J and Perry A, 'Assessment procedures for post-laryngectomy patients who desire surgical voice restoration', *Journal of Laryngology and Otology*, 100, 1985.

Darvill G, 'Rehabilitation – not just voice', Edels Y (ed), *Laryngectomy: Diagnosis to Rehabilitation*, Croom Helm, London, 1983.

Diedrich WM and Youngstrom HA, *Alaryngeal Speech*, Charles C. Thomas, Springfield, Illinois, 1966.

Diedrich WM and Youngstrom HA, *Alaryngeal Speech*, Charles C. Thomas, Springfield, Illinois, 1977.

Duguay M, 'Speech Problems of the Alaryngeal Speaker', Keith RL & Darley FL (eds), *Laryngectomee Rehabilitation*, College-Hill Press, Houston, 1986.

Edels Y, *Laryngectomy: Diagnosis to Rehabilitation*, Croom Helm, London, 1983.

Edwards N, 'Vocal Rehabilitation by External Vocal Fistula and Valved Prosthesis: Edwards Method', Shedd DP and Weinberg B (eds), *Surgical and Prosthetic Approaches to Speech Rehabilitation*, G K Hall Medical Publishers, Boston, 1980.

Faulkener WB, 'Objective esophageal changes due to psychic factors', *American Journal of Medical Sciences*, 200, 1940.

Gardner WH, *'Laryngectomee Speech and Rehabilitation'*, Charles C. Thomas, Springfield, Illinois, 1971.

Gates GA, Ryan W, Cooper JC, Lawlis GF, Cantu E, Hayashi T, Lauder E, Welch RW and Hearne E, 'Current Status of Laryngectomee Rehabilitation I. Results of Therapy', *American Journal of Otolaryngology*, 3, 1982.

Greene JS, 'Laryngectomy and its psychological implications', *NY State Journal of Medicine*, 47, 1947.

Greene MCL and Mathieson L, *The Voice and its Disorders*, 5th edn, Whurr Publishers Limited, London, 1989.

Hunt RB, 'Rehabilitation of the Laryngectomee', *Laryngoscope*, 74, 1964.

Hyman M, 'Evaluation of Speech Proficiency and Classification of Esophageal Speakers', University of Miami, Florida School of Medicine post-graduate class, 1957.

Keith RL, Shane HC, Coates HLC and Devine KD, *Looking Forward . . . A Guidebook for the Laryngectomee*, Thieme-Stratton Inc., New York, 1984.

Keith RL and Darley FL, *Laryngectomee Rehabilitation*, College-Hill Press, Houston, 1986.

King PS, Fowlks EW and Peirson GA, 'Rehabilitation and Adaptation of Laryngectomy Patients', *American Journal of Physical Medicine*, 47, 1968.

La Borwit LJ, 'The Development of an Inventory for the Assessment of Laryngectomee Rehabilitation' *XVth International Congress of Logopaedics and Phoniatrics*, Interlaken 1974, Kager, Basel, 1976.

Logemann JA, Fisher HB and Becker NG, 'Northwestern Otolaryngology Communication Profile', in Shedd DP and Weinberg B (eds), *Surgical and Prosthetic Approaches to Speech Rehabilitation*, GK Hall & Co, Boston, 1980.

MacCurtain FM, *Pharyngeal Factors Influencing Voice Quality*, University of London, 1981.

Murrils G, 'Pre- and early post-operative care of the Laryngectomee and Spouse', in Edels Y (ed), *Laryngectomy: Diagnosis to Rehabilitation*, Croom Helm, London, 1983.

Perry A, 'Assessment: what, why, how and when to measure social, physical, communication and psychological improvement', in Edels Y (ed), *Laryngectomy: Diagnosis to Rehabilitation*, Croom Helm, London, 1983.

Perry A, 'Assessing Surgical Voice Restoration following Laryngectomy', *College of Speech Therapists Bulletin*, No. 439, 1988a.

Perry A, 'Surgical voice restoration following laryngectomy: the tracheo-oesophageal fistula technique (Singer–Blom)', *British Journal of Disorders of Communication*, 23, 1, 1988b.

Perry A, Cheesman AD and Eden R, 'A Modification of the Blom–Singer Valve for Restoration of Voice after Laryngectomy', *Journal of Laryngology and Otology*, 96, 1982.

Perry A and Edels Y, 'Recent advances in the assessment of "failed" oesophageal speakers', *British Journal of Disorders of Communication*, 20, 3, 1985.

Perry A, Cheesman AD, McIvor J and Chalton R, 'A British experience of surgical voice restoration as a secondary procedure following total laryngectomy', *Journal of Laryngology and Otology*, 101, 1987.

Pitkin YN, 'Factors affecting psychologic adjustment in laryngectomised patients', *Annals of Otolaryngology*, 58, 38, 1953.

Richardson JL, 'Surgical and Radiological Effects upon the Development of Speech after Total Laryngectomy', *Annals of Otolaryngology*, 90, 1981.

Salmon SJ, 'Counselling of the laryngectomee and his spouse', paper presented at Laryngectomee Rehabilitation Seminar (Mayo Clinic), Honolulu, Hawaii, 1986a.

Salmon SJ, 'Methods of Air Intake for Esophageal Speech', paper presented at Laryngectomee Rehabilitation Seminar (Mayo Clinic), Honolulu, Hawaii, 1986b.

Salmon SJ, 'The Artificial Larynx', paper presented at Laryngectomee Rehabilitation Seminar (Mayo Clinic), Honolulu, Hawaii, 1986c.

Salmon SJ, 'Pre- and Post-operative Conferences with Laryngectomized and their Spouses', in Keith RL and Darley FL (eds), *Laryngectomee Rehabilitation*, College-Hill Press, Houston, 1986d.

Salmon SJ and Goldstein LP, *The Artificial Larynx Handbook*, Grune and Stratton, New York, 1978.

Samuel P and Adams FG, 'The Role of Oesophageal and Diaphragmatic Movements in Alaryngeal Speech', *Journal of Laryngology and Otolaryngology*, 90, 1976.

Seddon V, *After your Laryngectomy, a Guide for Patient and Family*, Lister Hospital, Stevenage, Herts (date not known).

Shanks J, 'An Initial Management Protocol for the New Laryngectomized Patient', paper presented at Laryngectomee Rehabilitation Seminar (Mayo Clinic), Honolulu, Hawaii, 1986a.

Shanks J, 'Essential for Alaryngeal Speech: Psychology and Physiology', in Keith RL and Darley FL (eds), *Laryngectomee Rehabilitation*, College-Hill Press, Houston, 1986b.

Shipp T, 'Frequency, Duration and Perceptual Measures in Relation to judgements of Alaryngeal Speech Acceptability', *Journal of Speech Hearing Research*, 10, 1967.

Simpson IC, Smith JCS and Gordon MT, 'Laryngectomy: the Influence of Muscle Reconstruction on the Mechanism of Oesophageal Voice Production', *Journal of Laryngology and Otology*, 86, 1972.

Singer MI and Blom ED, 'An Endoscopic Technique for Restoration of Voice after Laryngectomy', *Annals of Otology, Rhinology and Laryngology*, 89, 1980.

Singer MI and Blom ED, 'Selective myotomy for voice restoration after total laryngectomy', *Archives of Otolaryngology* 107, 1981.

Singer MI, Blom ED and Hamaker RC, 'Further Experience with Voice Restoration after Total Laryngectomy', *Archives of Otolaryngology*, 90, 1981.

Snidecor JC, 'Some Scientific Foundations for Voice Restoration', *Laryngoscope*, 85, 1975.

Stafford N, 'Surgical Adjustments to the Vocal Tract', paper presented at NALC Seminar, Royal Marsden Hospital, London, 1989.

Stoll B, 'Psychological Factors Determining the Success or Failure of the Rehabilitation Program of Laryngectomized Patients', *Annals of Otolaryngology*, 67, 1958.

Taub S and Bugner LH, 'Air Bypass Voice Prosthesis for Vocal Rehabilitation of Laryngectomees', *American Journal of Surgery*, 125, 1973.

Wepman JM, MacGahan JM, Rickard JC and Shelton WW, 'The Objective Measure of Progressive Esophageal Speech Development', *Journal of Speech and Hearing Disorders*, 18, 1953.

Wolfe RD, Olsen JE and Goldenberg DG, 'Rehabilitation of the Laryngectomee: the Role of the Distal Oesophageal Sphincter', *Laryngoscope*, 81, 1971.